Novel Imaging Techniques in Neurodegenerative and Movement Disorders

Editors

RATHAN M. SUBRAMANIAM
JORGE R. BARRIO

PET CLINICS

www.pet.theclinics.com

Consulting Editor
ABASS ALAVI

October 2013 • Volume 8 • Number 4

ELSEVIER

1600 John F. Kennedy Boulevard • Suite 1800 • Philadelphia, Pennsylvania, 19103-2899

http://www.theclinics.com

PET CLINICS Volume 8, Number 4
October 2013 ISSN 1556-8598, ISBN-13: 978-0-323-22735-3

Publisher: Adrianne-Brigido

© **2013 Elsevier Inc. All rights reserved.**

This periodical and the individual contributions contained in it are protected under copyright by Elsevier, and the following terms and conditions apply to their use:

Photocopying

Single photocopies of single articles may be made for personal use as allowed by national copyright laws. Permission of the Publisher and payment of a fee is required for all other photocopying, including multiple or systematic copying, copying for advertising or promotional purposes, resale, and all forms of document delivery. Special rates are available for educational institutions that wish to make photocopies for non-profit educational classroom use. For information on how to seek permission visit www.elsevier.com/permissions or call: (+44) 1865 843830 (UK)/(+1) 215 239 3804 (USA).

Derivative Works

Subscribers may reproduce tables of contents or prepare lists of articles including abstracts for internal circulation within their institutions. Permission of the Publisher is required for resale or distribution outside the institution. Permission of the Publisher is required for all other derivative works, including compilations and translations (please consult www.elsevier.com/permissions).

Electronic Storage or Usage

Permission of the Publisher is required to store or use electronically any material contained in this periodical, including any article or part of an article (please consult www.elsevier.com/permissions). Except as outlined above, no part of this publication may be reproduced, stored in a retrieval system or transmitted in any form or by any means, electronic, mechanical, photocopying, recording or otherwise, without prior written permission of the Publisher.

Notice

No responsibility is assumed by the Publisher for any injury and/or damage to persons or property as a matter of products liability, negligence or otherwise, or from any use or operation of any methods, products, instructions or ideas contained in the material herein. Because of rapid advances in the medical sciences, in particular, independent verification of diagnoses and drug dosages should be made. Although all advertising material is expected to conform to ethical (medical) standards, inclusion in this publication does not constitute a guarantee or endorsement of the quality or value of such product or of the claims made of it by its manufacturer.

PET Clinics (ISSN 1556-8598) is published quarterly by Elsevier Inc., 360 Park Avenue South, New York, NY 10010-1710. Months of issue are January, April, July, and October. Periodicals postage paid at New York, NY, and additional mailing offices. Subscription prices per year are $215.00 (US individuals), $309.00 (US institutions), $110.00 (US students), $244.00 (Canadian individuals), $345.00 (Canadian institutions), $134.00 (Canadian students), $260.00 (foreign individuals), $345.00 (foreign institutions), and $134.00 (foreign students). To receive student and resident rate, orders must be accompanied by name of affiliated institution, date of term, and the signature of program/residency coordinator on institution letterhead. Orders will be billed at individual rate until proof of status is received. Foreign air speed delivery is included in all Clinics subscription prices. All prices are subject to change without notice. POSTMASTER: Send address changes to PET Clinics, Elsevier Health Sciences Division, Subscription Customer Service, 3251 Riverport Lane, Maryland Heights, MO 63043. **Customer Service: 1-800-654-2452 (U.S. and Canada); 314-447-8871 (outside U.S. and Canada). Fax: 314-447-8029. E-mail: journalscustomerservice-usa@elsevier.com (for print support); journalsonlinesupport-usa@elsevier.com (for online support).**

Reprints. For copies of 100 or more of articles in this publication, please contact the Commercial Reprints Department, Elsevier Inc., 360 Park Avenue South, New York, NY 10010-1710. Tel.: 212-633-3874; Fax: 212-633-3820; E-mail: reprints@elsevier.com.

Printed in the United States of America.

Contributors

CONSULTING EDITOR

ABASS ALAVI, MD, PhD (Hon), DSc (Hon)
Professor of Radiology, Division of Nuclear
Medicine, Department of Radiology, University
of Pennsylvania School of Medicine, Hospital
of the University of Pennsylvania, Philadelphia,
Pennsylvania

EDITORS

RATHAN M. SUBRAMANIAM, MD, PhD, MPH
Russel H Morgan Department of Radiology and
Radiological Sciences, Johns Hopkins Medical
Institutions, Baltimore, Maryland

JORGE R. BARRIO, PhD
Professor of Biomedical Physics, Department
of Molecular and Medical Pharmacology,
David Geffen School of Medicine, University of
California Los Angeles, Los Angeles, California

AUTHORS

ROBERT M. COHEN, PhD, MD
Neuroscience Program, Graduate Division of
Biological and Medical Sciences, Department
of Psychiatry and Behavioral Neuroscience,
Emory University, Atlanta, Georgia

VIJAY DHAWAN, PhD
Investigator, Center for Neurosciences, The
Feinstein Institute for Medical Research,
Manhasset, New York

DORIS J. DOUDET, PhD
Professor, Department of Neurology,
University of British Columbia, Vancouver,
British Columbia, Canada

ALEXANDER DRZEZGA, MD
Professor, Head of Department, Department of
Nuclear Medicine, University Hospital Cologne,
Cologne, Germany

ANDREAS FELLGIEBEL, MD
Professor, Department of Psychiatry and
Psychotherapy, University Medical Center
Mainz, Mainz, Germany

SAMUEL FRANK, MD
Associate Professor of Neurology, Department
of Neurology, Boston University School of
Medicine, Boston, Massachusetts

FRANK JESSEN, MD
Professor, Department of Psychiatry, German
Center for Neurodegenerative Diseases
(DZNE), University of Bonn, Bonn, Germany

VLADIMIR KEPE, PhD
Researcher in Pharmacology, Department of
Molecular and Medical Pharmacology, David
Geffen School of Medicine, University of
California at Los Angeles, Los Angeles,
California

MICHAEL KLEINMAN, DO
Movement Disorders Fellow, Department of
Neurology, Boston University School of
Medicine, Boston, Massachusetts

HANNAH LOCKAU, MD
Department of Radiology, University Hospital
Cologne, Cologne, Germany

YILONG MA, PhD
Associate Investigator, Center for
Neurosciences, The Feinstein Institute for
Medical Research, Manhasset, New York

GUSTAVO MERCIER, MD, PhD
Department of Radiology, Boston University,
Boston, Massachusetts

PATRICK J. PELLER, MD
Department of Radiology, Mayo Clinic,
Rochester, Minnesota

SHICHUN PENG, PhD
Research Scientist, Center for Neurosciences,
The Feinstein Institute for Medical Research,
Manhasset, New York

RATHAN M. SUBRAMANIAM, MD, PhD, MPH
Russel H Morgan Department of Radiology
and Radiological Sciences, Johns
Hopkins Medical Institutions, Baltimore,
Maryland

DEVAKI SHILPA SURASI, MD
Department of Radiology, University of
Alabama, Birmingham, Alabama

ZSOLT SZABO, MD
Russel H Morgan Department of Radiology
and Radiological Sciences, Johns
Hopkins Medical Institutions, Baltimore,
Maryland

Contents

patient characteristics significantly increase mortality. Certain imaging modalities such as magnetic resonance imaging, transcranial ultrasound, and single-photon emission computed tomography can be useful in making diagnostic decisions in some cases of PD.

The clinical diagnosis of Parkinson disease (PD) is difficult, as several other neurodegenerative and basal ganglia disorders have similar clinical presentations. Dopamine transporter single-photon emission computed tomography has been proposed as possible diagnostic tool to help differentiate idiopathic PD from essential tremor and other disorders that present with parkinsonian symptoms. In addition, it is valuable in the diagnosis of dementia with Lewy bodies, differentiating it from other causes of dementia such as Alzheimer disease.

This article discusses the current use of PET imaging in the evaluation of dopamine function in Parkinson disease (PD). The article reviews the major radioligands targeting dopaminergic systems in patients with parkinsonian disorders. The primary objective is to show the novel clinical applications of molecular imaging in the diagnosis and assessment of motor and nonmotor symptoms in PD.

PET CLINICS

**DOWNLOAD
Free App!**

Review Articles
THE CLINICS

NOW AVAILABLE FOR YOUR iPhone and iPad

PROGRAM OBJECTIVE:

The goal of the PET Clinics is to keep practicing radiologists and radiology residents up to date with current clinical practice inpositron emission tomography by providing timely articles reviewing the state of the art in patient care.

TARGET AUDIENCE:

Practicing radiologists, radiology residents, and other health care professionals who provide patient care utilizing radiologic findings.

LEARNING OBJECTIVES

Upon completion of this activity, participants will be able to:

1. Discuss the epidemiology and clinical diagnosis of Alzheimer's disease.
2. Describe structural and functional Magnetic Resonance Imaging and Amyloid PET imaging of mild cognitive impairment and Alzheimer's disease.
3. Discuss the use of dopamine in PET imaging of Parkinson's disease and dopamine transporter imaging in Parkinson's disease and dementia.

ACCREDITATION

The Elsevier Office of Continuing Medical Education (EOCME) is accredited by the Accreditation Council for Continuing Medical Education (ACCME) to provide continuing medical education for physicians.

The EOCME designates this enduring material for a maximum of 15 *AMA PRA Category 1 Credit*(s)™. Physicians should claim only the credit commensurate with the extent of their participation in the activity.

All other health care professionals requesting continuing education credit for this enduring material will be issued a certificate of participation.

DISCLOSURE OF CONFLICTS OF INTEREST

The EOCME assesses conflict of interest with its instructors, faculty, planners, and other individuals who are in a position to control the content of CME activities. All relevant conflicts of interest that are identified are thoroughly vetted by EOCME for fair balance, scientific objectivity, and patient care recommendations. EOCME is committed to providing its learners with CME activities that promote improvements or quality in healthcare and not a specific proprietary business or a commercial interest.

The planning committee, staff, authors and editors listed below have identified no financial relationships or relationships to products or devices they or their spouse/life partner have with commercial interest related to the content of this CME activity:
Abass Alavi, MD, PhD (Hon), DSC (Hon); Jorge Barrio, PhD; Adrianne Brigido; Robert Cohen, MD, PhD; Nicole Congleton; Vijay Dhawan, PhD; Doris J. Doudet, PhD; Brynne Hunter; Frank Jessen, MD; Vladimir Kepe, PhD; Michael Kleinman, DO; Sandy Lavery; Hannah Lockau, MD; Yilong Ma, PhD; Jill McNair; Gustavo Mercier, MD, PhD; Mahalakshmi Narayanan; Shichun Peng, PhD; Devaki Shilpa Surasi, MD; Zsolt Szabo, MD, PhD.

The planning committee, staff, authors and editors listed below have identified financial relationships or relationships to products or devices they or their spouse/life partner have with commercial interest related to the content of this CME activity:
Alexander Drzezga, MD is on speakers bureau for GE Healthcare, Siemens Healthcare and Bayer Healthcare; is consultant/advisor for Piramal, Avid Pharmaceuticals/Lilly, and Bayer Healthcare.
Andreas Fellgiebel, MD is a consultant/advisor for GE Healthcare, Lilly and Genzyme, a Sanofi Company; has a research grant from Shire; and is on speakers bureau for Genzyme, a Sanofi Company.
Samuel Frank, MD is a consultant/advisor for Merz; has a research grant with Auspex.
Patrick J. Peller, MD is on speakers bureau for Eli Lilly and Company.
Rathan M. Subramaniam, MD, PhD, MPH, MClinEd, FRANZCR, MRSNZ is on speakers bureau for Eli Lilly: Amyloid PET speaker program.

UNAPPROVED/OFF-LABEL USE DISCLOSURE

The EOCME requires CME faculty to disclose to the participants:

1. When products or procedures being discussed are off-label, unlabelled, experimental, and/or investigational (not US Food and Drug Administration (FDA) approved); and
2. Any limitations on the information presented, such as data that are preliminary or that represent ongoing research, interim analyses, and/or unsupported opinions. Faculty may discuss information about pharmaceutical agents that is outside of FDA-approved labelling. This information is intended solely for CME and is not intended to promote off-label use of these medications. If you have any questions, contact the medical affairs department of the manufacturer for the most recent prescribing information.

TO ENROLL

To enroll in the Sleep Medicines Clinic Continuing Medical Education program, call customer service at 1-800-654-2452 or sign up online at http://www.theclinics.com/home/cme. The CME program is available to subscribers for an additional annual fee of USD 126.

METHOD OF PARTICIPATION

In order to claim credit, participants must complete the following:

1. Complete enrolment as indicated above.
2. Read the activity.
3. Complete the CME Test and Evaluation. Participants must achieve a score of 70% on the test. All CME Tests and Evaluations must be completed online.

CME INQUIRIES/SPECIAL NEEDS

For all CME inquiries or special needs, please contact elsevierCME@elsevier.com.

Epidemiology and Clinical Diagnosis: Alzheimer Disease

Robert M. Cohen, PhD, MD

KEYWORDS

- Alzheimer - Dementia - Amyloid - Tau - Neurodegeneration - Apolipoprotein

KEY POINTS

- Alzheimer disease (AD) is the sixth leading cause of death in the United States. Incidence rates increase exponentially from age 65 years on.
- Onset of AD before age 60 (EOAD) and at 65 years and older (LOAD) share similar postmortem findings, but vary in their clinical presentations.
- Therapeutic disappointments, the complex genetics of LOAD, and new findings related to regional progression of pathology have led to new hypotheses that emphasize either the vulnerability of the aging brain with respect to stress, or a neuron-to-neuron transmission process similar to what is observed in prion disorders.
- Mounting evidence suggests that the initial physiologic changes (preclinical phase) that place the brain on the pathway to LOAD occur at least 20 years before dementia symptoms appear. This initial preclinical phase is followed by a phase whereby cognitive impairment, but no functional impairment, is present (mild cognitive impairment), which is then followed by the third phase of dementia.
- Diagnosis of AD has primarily been one of exclusion of all other causes of reversible and irreversible dementia. Overlapping clinical presentations of diseases causing neurodegeneration, however, create challenges for accurate diagnosis.
- Use of clinical magnetic resonance and PET imaging modalities increase the specificity of diagnosis. Several new promising experimental approaches are discussed in other articles elsewhere in this issue.

THE NUMBERS

The unintended consequence of medicine's success in prolonging life, combined with the aging population of industrialized nations, has been an increase in the prevalence of Alzheimer disease (AD), by far the most common form of dementia and one in which age is the most important risk factor. With an already unprecedented 35 million people in the world suffering from AD and with the expectation in the near future that someone will be joining these ranks every 35 seconds, these numbers are expected to increase dramatically,[1] thus establishing dementia not only as the sixth leading cause of death in the United States but also one of the most costly diseases worldwide.

To understand why this is the case, one need only to recall that at the end of the nineteenth century life expectancy was in the 40s, a consequence of which is that of all the people who have ever lived to age 65, more than half are now alive. Next, it is important to examine how people die in industrialized nations. Three major pathways account for most deaths and reinforces why AD, if not currently, will shortly become the most costly of all illnesses. Although 20% of individuals die of cancer with a peak at age 65 years, this illness is generally associated with a relatively quick

Neuroscience Program, Graduate Division of Biological and Medical Sciences, Department of Psychiatry and Behavioral Neuroscience, Emory University, 101 Woodruff Circle, Suite WMB4003, Atlanta, GA 30322, USA
E-mail address: Robert.m.cohen@emory.edu

PET Clin 8 (2013) 391–405
http://dx.doi.org/10.1016/j.cpet.2013.08.001
1556-8598/13/$ – see front matter © 2013 Elsevier Inc. All rights reserved.

downward path from highly functional individuals to poor functioning and then death. Another 25% of deaths are attributable to heart and lung failure that peaks at around 75 years of age. These individuals have a gradual decline punctuated by dips in function, followed by recoveries that asymptote short of their level of function that preceded each dip. However, for the rest of the population death follows a prolonged period of frailty and dementia.

Finally, although incidence rates may differ among Asian, African, African American, and Hispanic ethnic groups, all share similar exponentially related increases in incidence with age, resulting in prevalence rates of dementia rising from less than 5% of the population younger than 65 years to, in some studies, prevalence rates that approach 50% after the age of 85 and with at least 50% of all dementias occurring after the age of 65 attributable to AD.[2] This trend takes on added significance when one considers data from the US Census Bureau establishing the oldest of old as the fastest-growing age group in the United States by percentage, with 51,000 Americans already having surpassed the century milestone. Of importance is that recent studies, in contrast to earlier studies, have not indicated any curtailment of incidence rates at any advanced age, suggesting that an individual having reached a certain age would be unlikely to subsequently suffer from AD, leading to the very real possibility that at some point, should an individual live long enough, that person will eventually develop AD. Some solace, however, may be taken from evidence that the phenotypic expression of AD in those older than 85 years appears to be relatively mild while also making the clinical diagnosis of AD correspondingly difficult.

PATHOPHYSIOLOGY OF AD

Although the cardinal pathologic features of AD, namely the presence of extracellular senile plaques and intracellular neurofibrillary tangles (NFT) at postmortem, were established more than a century ago, it was not until the 1980s that an understanding of the proteins that are the major components of each of these were determined to be β-amyloid and hyperphosphorylated tau. The findings provided the basis for rapid progress beginning with the discovery that β-amyloid, primarily consisting of $A\beta_{1-40}$ and $A\beta_{1-42}$, was the product of aberrant processing of amyloid precursor protein (APP) by β-secretases and γ-secretases (**Fig. 1**). Mutations in the 3 genes APP, Presenilin 1 (PSEN1), and Presenilin 2 (PSEN2), the latter 2 genes coding for proteins that are components of the multisubunit γ-secretase, were soon discovered to be the causes of early-onset AD (EOAD; age of onset before 60 years) in families showing autosomal dominant inheritance. Each of the mutations was found to increase the cellular production of aggregation-prone products of APP processing that are toxic to cells (ie, $A\beta_{1-40}$ and $A\beta_{1-42}$), solidifying the amyloid cascade hypothesis.[3]

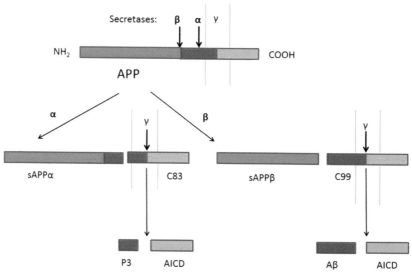

Fig. 1. Processing of amyloid precursor protein (APP). Aβ is formed by the sequential action of β- and γ-secretases. The competing alternative pathway through α- and γ-secretases does not produce toxic products. Vertical lines depict cell membrane. Carboxy-terminal end of APP is inside cell. AICD, APP intracellular domain.

AMYLOID CASCADE HYPOTHESIS

In brief, the hypothesis identifies the toxic products of an abnormal processing of APP as leading to the formation of abnormal forms of tau, synapse dysfunction, and neuronal death that form the basis of the clinical symptoms of both EOAD and late forms of AD (LOAD; age of onset 65 years and older). Over the years, the particular nature of the aggregates that are most harmful have changed, with the current belief that soluble oligomers are the chief offending forms. The hypothesis relies heavily on viewing LOAD through the prism of EOAD, a not unreasonable approach given the many shared pathologic features of the two disorders. Because evidence in favor of an increase in abnormal APP processing as an initiating event for LOAD has been in short supply, variants of the amyloid cascade hypothesis for LOAD have arisen. These proposals have included extracellular milieus favoring aggregation (eg, metals), and difficulties clearing β-amyloid from the brain. In this regard it is notable that brain clearance of β-amyloid can occur through peptidase breakdown, microglia uptake, and low-density lipoprotein receptor-related protein 1 (LRP-1)-mediated endothelial transport. In contrast to exit, β-amyloid entry to the brain is mediated through the receptor for advanced glycation end products (RAGE).[4] The asymmetric transport mechanisms for entry and exit pathways allows for the possibility of changes in intracellular or extracellular components to favor entry or exit. For example, oxygen stress appears to reduce LRP-1 capacity while increasing RAGE capacity.[5]

Although autosomal dominant mutations account for less than 1% of AD cases, the amyloid cascade hypothesis led to the development of animal models of AD and has been the basis of most experimental treatments of AD: inhibiting β-secretases and γ-secretases; enhancing a nontoxic competing pathway for APP processing by enhancing α-secretase activity; blocking $A\beta_{1-40}$ and $A\beta_{1-42}$ aggregation; promoting disaggregation of Aβ oligomers; increasing clearance of toxic products of the APP processing pathway, including enhancement of enzymes that degrade β-amyloid or facilitating transport of Aβ from brain; and passive and active vaccine approaches targeting β-amyloid. The latter has been the object of the most clinical trials. Unfortunately, despite evidence of some success at lessening brain amyloid with vaccine strategies, clinical success has eluded all approaches.[6]

These therapeutic disappointments, together with findings that EOAD and LOAD can have differences in their clinical presentations and rates of progression, that mutations in the tau gene (MAPT) can also produce dementia, and that abnormal tau regional brain distribution does not parallel amyloid deposition but has a stronger association with degree of cognitive impairment,[7] have led to a questioning of the underlying assumption of the amyloid cascade hypothesis for LOAD; that is, that LOAD shares the same fundamental cause as autosomal dominant forms of EOAD. Two very different paradigms have been proposed to fill the perceived void. These paradigms question not only whether abnormal APP processing is at the heart of LOAD, but even whether the observed pathologic situation reflects the actual causes of the disease or simply innocent bystanders (ie, damage created by the causes of the disease), or in fact evidence of repair that has, unfortunately, not been sufficient to protect the individual from developing AD.

STRESS IN THE AGING BRAIN

The first of these 2 new paradigms is based on the most important risk factor for LOAD: age and the changes with age that are likely to make older neurons particularly vulnerable to stressful events.[8] These age-related changes include decreases in the efficacy of systems involved in surveillance and fixing of misfolded proteins,[9] protection against free radicals, mitochondrial function that can result in increases in free radicals,[10] central nervous system immune system function,[11] and regional cerebral blood flow. The aging brain faced with an insult, for example, a drop in cerebral perfusion or exposure of the brain to trauma, produces a chronic rather than a discrete neuroinflammatory response. The brain milieu, which now includes neuroinflammatory cytokines and activated microglia and astrocytes, interacts with neurons to induce a feed-forward cycle. The feed-forward cycle is depicted as eventually producing a radical change in cell state that includes changes in metabolism akin to what is observed in cancer or cells undergoing growth, which includes changes in cell-cycle proteins and proteins involved in remodeling of synapses, spines, and dendrites, in metabolic pathways designed to support pro-growth (Warburg effect)[12] and an increase in amyloid production and abnormal tau. Eventually these adaptations to stress fail, leading to greater cell dysfunction and death.

NEURON-TO-NEURON TRANSMISSION

The second new paradigm has as its basis prion disorders. In these disorders abnormally folded proteins are responsible for cell dysfunction, and are transmitted from the initiating neuron to other neurons along the efferent pathway of those cells.[13] Although in contrast to prions there is no evidence of direct transmission of AD among humans, animal models and findings from post-mortem studies lend credence to the analogy. For example, injection of aggregated amyloid collected postmortem has been demonstrated to lead to amyloidosis when injected directly into the cerebral cortex of rodents, not only in the areas directly injected but also into neighboring areas receiving efferents. More recently even parenteral injections into mice of such materials, presumably through macrophage transport, have led to vascular amyloidosis as well as cerebral amyloidosis.[14] Postmortem studies in humans have, at least, in typical AD, observed a consistent pattern of regional brain involvement whereby abnormal tau is first observed in the entorhinal cortex, only subsequently observed in the adjacent areas of subiculum and then hippocampus, and from there to the limbic system, before spreading to the neocortex. However, new evidence has emerged from several groups to suggest that decades before the age that tau can be found in the cortex, abnormal tau accumulation is visible in norepinephrine cells of the locus coeruleus of healthy individuals in their third decade of life.[15] The presence of long axons on these neurons that do not receive substantial myelination have spurred speculation that this may be the cause of their particular vulnerability as well as the vulnerability of other neurons to AD pathology, as efferents from these neurons are not only directed to the medial temporal cortex, but have a broad distribution across both limbic and neocortical areas.

Although each of these paradigms differs in emphasis, there is considerable overlap between them. Moreover, it may be that patients with clinically diagnosed AD, while actually having different initial causes, develop the key pathologic features that warrant a pathologic diagnosis of AD. The possibility of different initial causes could in part explain that while there is a "classic" or typical clinical presentation of LOAD, there are several variant clinical presentations as described subsequently.

EPIDEMIOLOGY

Although geographic distribution of disease has often shed light on causative agents of disease, this has not been especially true with respect to AD, as the relative incidence of AD in various parts of the world is similar. Where there are small differences, it is difficult to rule out methodological differences that may have contributed to observed ethnic and national variations. However, the study of selected populations, families, and twins has led to a better understanding of the degree of genetic in comparison with "environmental" contributions to risk and age of onset of AD and, perhaps most importantly, has contributed to the discovery of specific genetic and nongenetic factors. The latter have contributed greatly to our understanding of the LOAD disease process. While these studies have confirmed age as the preeminent risk factor for LOAD, it is likely that both genetic factors and environmental factors contribute to the risk and age of onset of both EOAD and LOAD. Studies of identical twins, for example, suggest that hereditability is somewhere between 60% and 80% for LOAD.

GENETICS

With respect to genetic factors for risk and age of onset of LOAD, variation in the apolipoprotein E (APOE) gene is known to have the greatest impact. The human APOE gene has 3 alleles: APOE-ε2, APOE-ε3, and APOE-ε4. Individuals carrying a single APOE-ε4 allele have 3 times the risk of developing AD and develop it earlier than those with the APOE-ε3 allele, the most common allele, and those with 2 APOE-ε4 alleles have a 9- to 15-fold increased risk. By contrast, inheritance of an APOE-ε2 allele, the rarest allele, confers some degree of protection. It was the initial finding of the presence of the APOE protein in amyloid plaques that led to the discovery of this important genetic risk factor. Despite this high odds ratio, the APOE gene only accounts for 23% of LOAD hereditability, and this has led to concerted efforts to determine additional genes associated with AD risk.[16]

Several additional common alleles have been found to contribute to AD risk but, disappointingly, they each make only a small contribution to risk, increasing the odds of developing AD risk by between 1.2 and 1.5. The genes identified include (among many others) SORL1, PICALM, TOMM40, GSK3β, CR1, and CLU. In many instances the products of these genes appear to either play a role in the production of Aβ, interact with Aβ, or are related to tau or to immune function. SORL1 is important for the processing of APP in the endosomal cell compartment and PICALM for the transport of APP across the endothelium; TOMM40, located on the outer mitochondrial membrane, interacts with APP. GSL3β phosphorylates tau, CR1 is a negative regulator of the complement cascade, and CLU, a lipoprotein, is highly expressed with stress and can act as a chaperone of importance in Aβ formation.[16,17]

Simulation studies suggest that 100 loci with allele frequencies similar to the aforementioned genes would be required to reach discriminative accuracy of 70% for the diagnosis of AD.[16] The complex genetics for LOAD contrast with the autosomal dominant genetics of EOAD, although there is some evidence that rare genetic variants in APP, PSEN1, and PSEN2 as well as many other genes may influence the risk for LOAD.[17] Although autosomal dominant inheritance of EOAD is emphasized here, it is notable that some 40% of EOAD patients do not have multiple members of the family affected and are characterized as sporadic cases, but may have underlying autosomal recessive causes.[18]

NONGENETIC FACTORS

Diabetes, depression, high cholesterol and high body mass index, traumatic brain injury in mid-life, smoking, occupational exposure to pesticides, and (possibly) lower education have been associated with higher risk or earlier age of onset, whereas increased physical activity, fish consumption or long-chain omega-3 fatty acid supplements, and participation in cognitively stimulating activities including social engagement (marital status, size and quality of social network, level of social activities and living arrangements) appear to be associated with lower risk or later age of onset.[19] Not surprisingly, given the overlap in the risk factors for cardiovascular disease and LOAD, risk factors for vascular disease and stroke are associated with cognitive impairment and LOAD, with approximately 40% of patients with LOAD having severe cardiovascular disease and almost all patients with severe cardiovascular disease showing concurrent AD pathology. While cerebrovascular disease is itself associated with cognitive impairment and severity of LOAD, intracranial atherosclerosis, independent of cerebral infarction (even microscopic) and aortic or cardiac atherosclerosis, appears to be a significant risk factor for the development of LOAD. This finding is important in that there is only a weak correlation between intracranial atherosclerosis and the severity of coronary and aortic atherosclerosis and carotid bifurcation atherosclerosis, whereas hypertension is the principal risk factor for intracranial atherosclerosis. The basis of this association is not known. Possibilities include a common cause for both; for example, a direct effect of $A\beta$ or oxidative stress, white matter disease, inflammation, or an association between large-vessel abnormality and small-vessel endothelium dysfunction.

Epidemiology studies demonstrating that mid-life use of nonsteroidal anti-inflammatories reduced the risk of AD[20] helped initiate a broad range of studies that have demonstrated the importance of the immune system in AD pathology, which up to that time had received scant investigation. More recent studies have shown that patients given intravenous immunoglobulin (IVIg),[21] most often to treat immune deficiencies, lymphomas, thrombocytopenia, or chronic inflammatory diseases such as demyelinating polyneuritis, appear to be at lower risk of developing LOAD. IVIg is currently being investigated as a therapeutic agent in the treatment of AD, as is a broad range of treatments aimed at optimizing the immune system.

CLINICAL DIAGNOSIS OF AD

Recognizing that different dementias can have overlapping clinical presentations, the initial set of guidelines for the diagnosis of AD promulgated by a joint working group of the National Institute for Neurological and Communicative Disorders and Stroke and the Alzheimer's Disease and Related Disorders Association (NINCDS-ADRDA) recognized the difference between the clinical diagnosis of AD and the pathologic diagnosis of AD. As in a previous, but similar version of the definition of AD, given in the *Diagnostic and Statistical Manual of Mental Disorders* (**Box 1**), the 1984 guidelines

---

Box 1
DSM-IV diagnostic criteria for AD

Multiple cognitive deficits

  Short- and long-term memory impairment

    AND one or more of the following:

      Aphasia (language)

      Apraxia (impaired ability to carry out familiar tasks)

      Agnosia (failure to recognize familiar objects)

      Disturbances in executive function (planning, organizing, abstract thinking)

Gradual onset, significant functional (social or occupational) impairment, and continuous decline

Decline from a previously higher level of function

Exclusion of other possible causes

  No evidence of delirium (or metabolic-toxic encephalopathy characterized by fluctuating levels of awareness)

Abbreviation: DSM-IV, *Diagnostic and Statistical Manual of Mental Disorders* (4th edition, text revised).

(NINCDS-ADRDA criteria, **Box 2**) recognized that the ultimate diagnosis of AD was a neuropathologic one that could only be made at postmortem and yet, given the impracticality of biopsy, it was important to establish guidelines for making at least a tentative clinical diagnosis of AD. Essentially the guidelines required the development of memory impairment and 1 or more of aphasia, apraxia, agnosia, or executive functioning (planning, organizing, sequencing, abstracting, and so forth), each of which was sufficiently severe as to cause significant decline from the individual's previous level of social or occupational functioning. However, they also required that the decline in function is not exclusively present when the individual is delirious, or when mental disorders or other non–AD-associated etiologic organic factors can reasonably account for the change (eg, hypothyroidism, normal-pressure hydrocephalus). The reader may well recognize that with the exceptions of requiring the presence of memory impairment as 1 of the 2 categories of cognitive impairment and excluding patients with non–AD-associated organic factors, these criteria are essentially those for the diagnosis of dementia. At the time laboratory data, as they still do today, were considered important exclusionary criteria in establishing these other, sometimes reversible causes of

dementia. It has been generally accepted that clinicians can achieve a success rate approximating 80% sensitivity and specificity of about 70% when measured against postmortem diagnosis.

CURRENT GUIDELINES

In the nearly 30 years that have elapsed from the first appearance of these guidelines, the depth and breadth of our understanding of the pathophysiologic underpinnings of AD has dramatically expanded, as have our abilities to measure an individual's phenotype and genotype. Imaging now allows for the direct measurement of brain structure and, to a great extent, brain function, making it possible for us to infer neuronal loss and network dysfunction. Advances in genotyping allow us to, at least to some degree, assess genotype risk as well as, when called for, directly determine mutations that convey 100% risk. Furthermore, through the advent of new PET tracers and our improving capacity to measure biomarkers reliably in the cerebrospinal fluid (CSF), we can infer the presence of amyloid plaques and NFT, the pathognomonic AD brain lesions. Yet despite these advances, the clinical diagnosis and even to some extent the postmortem diagnosis of AD has become muddied as our awareness grows of the insidious nature of the disease, the multiple challenges that the aging brain is confronted with, and the knowledge of shared pathology with other dementias (dementia with Lewy bodies, vascular dementia, the behavioral variant of frontotemporal dementia, and primary progressive aphasia), and the discordant clinical and pathologic findings found in some individuals (eg, healthy individuals with substantial amyloid loads, individuals with mild cognitive impairment [MCI]) and others with nonamnestic dementia presentations (eg, posterior cortical atrophy and logopenic primary progressive aphasia) that meet the requirements for the postmortem diagnosis of AD. Even patients presenting with prominent motor symptoms can have pathologically confirmed AD. For example, as many as 40% of individuals presenting as corticobasal syndromes are shown to have AD pathology and many patients meeting postmortem criteria for AD are found to have Lewy bodies, particularly in limbic areas. This new knowledge has led to a renewed interest in the examination of how AD is defined. For example, should AD be defined on the basis of a cognitive profile, molecular or genotype determinants, specific pathologic findings, or on some combination of these? Is there an AD spectrum?

As a result of this new knowledge (as incomplete as it was and still is), in 2011 the National Institute

---

Box 2
NINCDS-ADRDA criteria

Probable AD

  Deficits in 2 or more cognitive domains

  Progressive worsening of memory and other cognitive domains

  No disturbance of consciousness

  Onset between 40 and 90 years of age

  Absence of other systemic disorders

  Impaired activities of daily life

  Associated behavioral abnormalities

Possible AD

  Dementia in the absence of other causes

  Presence of variations in

    Onset

    Presentation

    Clinical course

Uncertain/Unlikely AD

  Sudden onset

  Focal neurologic findings

  Early seizure or gait disturbances

on Aging Alzheimer's Association Workgroup promulgated a new set of diagnostic guidelines for AD. In essence the guidelines call for establishing the presence of dementia as already defined and then subsetting those with dementia into the clinical classifications of either Possible or Probable AD dementia, with a third and fourth research classification of Probable or Possible AD dementia with evidence of AD pathophysiologic process. **Box 3** is adapted, with minor modifications, from McKhann and colleagues.[22] Specifically with respect to making the diagnosis of dementia, emphasis is given to both cognitive (memory: getting lost in familiar situations, repetitive questions or stories, placing objects in odd places, executive function: risky behavior, inability to manage finances or plan for sequential activities; visuospatial: inability to recognize objects, or people, or not knowing how to use common objects, eg, a can opener; language: difficulties with reading or writing, or speaking) and neuropsychiatric symptoms (personality changes that can include rapid

---

Box 3
Diagnosis of dementia

Probable AD:

1. Inclusion Criteria:

    a. Onset of symptoms occurs over months to years with clear-cut progression of cognitive deficits as established by either report or observation. Symptoms should be based on the presence of one of the following cognitive profiles: an amnestic presentation (the most common) in which deficits in the learning and recall of information are prominent, and a nonamnestic presentation in which language (word finding), visuospatial (object agnosia, face recognition, simultanagnosia, and/ or alexia), or executive dysfunction (impaired reasoning, judgment and problem solving) are most prominent.

2. Exclusion Criteria:

    a. Evidence of substantial cerebrovascular disease as suggested by a history of stroke or the presence of multiple or extensive infarcts or severe white matter hyperintensity. Evidence should predate onset or worsening of dementia symptoms.

    b. The presence of core features of other dementias not typically associated with AD: for example, dementia with Lewy bodies; early onset of balance problems and/or visual hallucinations; behavioral variant frontotemporal dementia; early onset of dramatic changes in behavior predating obvious memory impairment; the semantic and nonfluent/agrammatic variants of primary progressive aphasia (PPA); prominent language impairments predating prominent memory impairment.

    c. Evidence of other neurologic or non-neurologic disorders that could account for the symptoms (eg, substantial exposure to heavy metals; Wernicke-Korsakoff syndrome, Wilson disease)

    d. Concurrent use of medication that could account for a substantial component of the symptoms listed under Inclusion Criteria.

Possible AD Dementia:

1. Inclusion Criteria:

    Meets criteria for AD dementia but has either:

    a. Atypical course with sudden onset of symptoms, or insufficient historical evidence to determine temporal pattern of onset or lacking objective evidence of progressive decline.

    b. Etiology is obfuscated by presence of Exclusion Criteria under Probable AD.

Possible AD dementia with evidence of the AD pathophysiological process is reserved for individuals who meet the criteria for a non-AD dementia, but who either show biomarker evidence of AD pathophysiology or meet the neuropathologic criteria for AD.

Dementia unlikely to be due to AD is reserved for individuals who, though meeting criteria for probable or possible AD, have strong evidence for an alternative diagnosis that rarely or never is associated with the presence of AD dementia.

Adapted from McKhann GM, Knopman DS, Chertkow H, et al. The diagnosis of dementia due to Alzheimer's disease: recommendations from the National Institute on Aging-Alzheimer's Association workgroups on diagnostic guidelines for Alzheimer's disease. Alzheimers Dement 2011;7:263–9; with permission.

changes in mood that can include irritability, agitation, loss of motivation, inability to sustain attention, new obsessions and compulsions, socially unacceptable behaviors suggesting both errors in judgment and disinhibition) as established by a combination of history taking, generally to be obtained from both the patient and a knowledgable informant, and objective cognitive assessment, such as obtained through a mental status examination and more extensive, but not compulsory neuropsychological testing. Having determined the presence of dementia, an algorithm for determining that a patient meets these new criteria for Probable or Possible AD is provided in **Fig. 2**. **Fig. 3** depicts an algorithm for making the determination of Possible or Probable AD along with the qualifying phrase with atypical or etiologically mixed presentation.

The new guidelines propose the use of several additional qualifying phrases to those patients categorized as having Probable AD dementia (**Fig. 4**) as well as Possible AD (**Fig. 5**). The qualifying phrase "with increased level of certainty" can be added to the designation of Probable AD dementia when there is documented evidence of cognitive decline from both informants and cognitive testing. The phrase "in a carrier of a causative AD genetic mutation" is given to those individuals meeting the criteria for Probable AD dementia who have a genetic mutation in APP, PSEN1, or PSEN2. The phrase "with evidence of the AD pathophysiologic process" is added when there is evidence for the presence of biomarkers reflective of the pathophysiologic processes that are believed to underpin the AD clinical profile. These biomarkers include magnetic resonance (MR) imaging evidence of disproportionate atrophy in the medial, basal, and lateral temporal cortex and medial parietal cortex, disproportionately decreased cerebral metabolism in temporoparietal cortex as appreciated on an ^{18}F-fluorodeoxyglucose (FDG) PET scan (**Fig. 6**), evidence of increased CSF total tau (t-tau) (>300% of normal) and/or phosphorylated tau (p-tau), and decreased $A\beta_{1-42}$ (<50% of normal) (**Fig. 7**). Although not mentioned in the guidelines by McKhann and colleagues,[22] a reduced ratio of Aβ/tau and unequivocal evidence of brain amyloid accumulations should probably be added to the list, which would qualify a patient to be given the added qualifier of "with evidence of the AD pathophysiologic process." Finally, there is

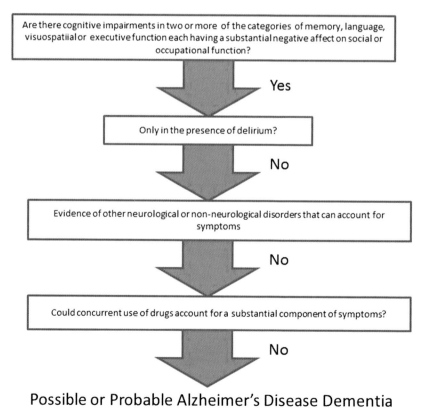

Are there cognitive impairments in two or more of the categories of memory, language, visuospatiial or executive function each having a substantial negative affect on social or occupational function?

Yes

Only in the presence of delirium?

No

Evidence of other neurological or non-neurological disorders that can account for symptoms

No

Could concurrent use of drugs account for a substantial component of symptoms?

No

Possible or Probable Alzheimer's Disease Dementia

Fig. 2. Algorithm for determination of possible or probable Alzheimer disease (AD).

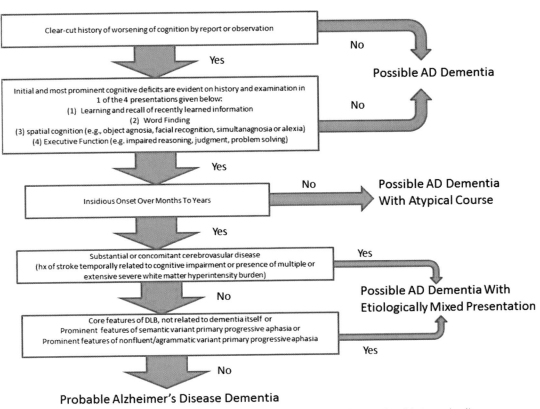

Fig. 3. Algorithm for deciding between possible or probable AD. DLB, dementia with Lewy bodies.

the category of possible AD dementia with evidence of the AD pathologic process for patients who receive a clinical diagnosis of a non-AD dementia but meet neuropathologic criteria for AD dementia or test positive for the 2 categories of AD biomarkers; that is, those reflecting amyloid abnormality as well as that of typical AD neuronal loss. The approach to these qualifiers is illustrated in **Figs. 4** and **5**.

Fig. 6 illustrates the type of FDG PET scan that the new criteria would agree supports the pathophysiologic AD process. **Fig. 7** illustrates how Aβ and t-tau or p-tau levels could be used to provide additional evidence of pathophysiologic process of AD by either using a ratio of Aβ/tau or independently determining either decreased Aβ (~50% of normal) or increased t-tau (300% of normal) or both, providing even more supportive evidence.

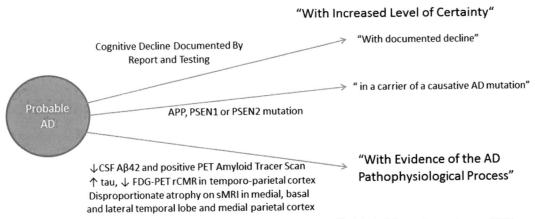

Fig. 4. Probable AD dementia qualifiers. CSF, cerebrospinal fluid; FDG, ^{18}F-labeled fluorodeoxyglucose; PSEN, presenilin; rCMR, regional cerebral metabolic rate; sMRI, structural magnetic resonance imaging.

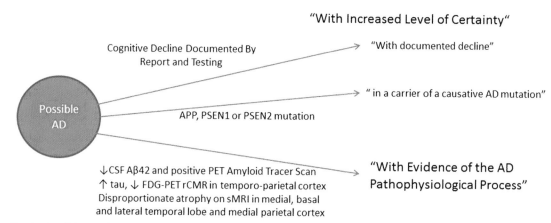

Fig. 5. Possible AD dementia qualifiers.

MILD COGNITIVE IMPAIRMENT

AD patients usually pass through a stage (MCI) when objective and subjective cognitive impairment can be appreciated, but when activities of daily living remain essentially normal. MCI patients can be subdivided into those who demonstrate a predominant memory component of cognitive impairment (amnestic MCI or aMCI) and those for whom other areas of cognitive impairment are

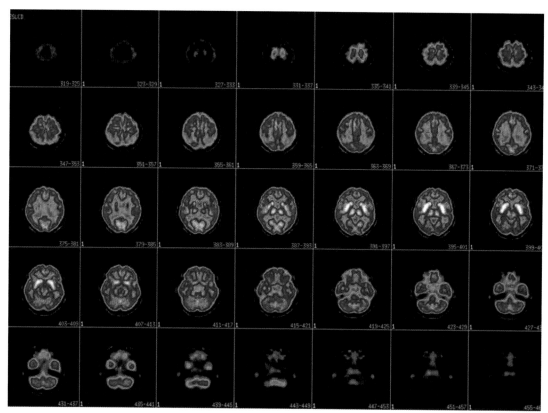

Fig. 6. Prototypical ^{18}F-FDG PET scan of an AD patient demonstrating prominent reduced regional cerebral metabolism in the parietotemporal cortices in the presence of reduced frontal cortical metabolism. Reductions are symmetric. Basal ganglia, thalamus, and primary motor and sensory cortical regions are spared. Axial slices from top (*upper left*) to bottom of brain (*lower right*). White and yellow represent highest metabolic rates and blue the lowest rates.

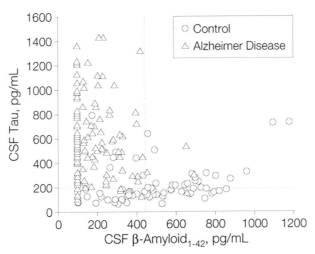

Fig. 7. Scatterplot of cerebrospinal fluid total tau and $A\beta_{1-42}$ of healthy controls and AD patients. Vertical and horizontal lines illustrate ideal cutoff points for discriminating healthy controls from AD patients in this particular sample and with this particular assay. (*From* Sunderland T, Linker G, Mirza N, et al. Decreased beta-amyloid$_{1-42}$ and increased tau levels in cerebrospinal fluid of patients with Alzheimer disease. JAMA 2003;289(16):2094–103; with permission.)

more prominent (ie, a nonamnestic variety or naMCI).[23] Although patients from both categories may progress to develop AD, aMCI patients have a higher risk of transitioning to AD. Moreover, patients who demonstrate greater medial temporal lobe atrophy, hippocampal atrophy, lower medial temporal lobe metabolism, or greater cognitive impairment are at greater risk for conversion. The new MCI category of MCI-AD with the above core clinical criteria supplemented with biomarker information akin to the use of biomarkers in AD has been recommended by the National Institute on Aging AD Working Group. MCI-AD is considered of high likelihood when $A\beta$ is low and tau is high, and of intermediate likelihood with low $A\beta$ or high tau.

As postmortem AD findings strongly suggest progression from the medial temporal lobe with spread to other brain regions (ie, lateral temporal lobe, parieto-occipital cortex, and frontal lobe structures), how is it possible that AD patients can follow a nonamnestic MCI pathway? It would seem that there are atypical AD presentations. It has long been recognized that some patients with confirmed AD postmortem pathology started with a clinical picture in which abnormal visual-spatial deficits including, most dramatically, cortical blindness, were the initial symptoms, with other patients showing evidence of prominent early symptoms primarily affecting language. These atypical variants demonstrating focal clinical presentations generally progress more slowly and are often mistakenly diagnosed as Lewy body dementia, prion diseases, corticobasal degeneration, one of the frontal temporal lobe dementias such as primary progressive aphasia, or a posterior cortical atrophy variant that involves occipital and parietal cortices leading to clinical symptoms that may include visual agnosia or acalculia, alexia or agraphia, or simultanagnosia.[24]

PRECLINICAL AD

As there is substantial evidence that AD pathology begins at least 20 years before the onset of clinical symptoms and the majority of MCI patients who will convert to AD will do so by 5 years, there has to be a pre-MCI period during which the pathophysiologic process of AD is present in the absence of any clinical manifestations.[25] Theoretically patients at some time during this pre-MCI or preclinical period begin to accumulate β-amyloid in the brain, and some years later would test positive with amyloid-dependent tracers. This period might even be further subdivided, depending on more subtle changes in cognition shown by PET studies of regional cerebral metabolism or other functional imaging procedures that currently go undetected in studies of group differences, but might well be detected with within-subject designs.

THE PRACTICING PHYSICIAN

Although the aforementioned algorithms may prove most helpful to researchers, the practicing clinician should benefit from further discussion of which diseases may be mistaken for AD dementia. First and foremost, it is important to distinguish delirium from dementia. Although abnormal functioning of almost any organ and infection can lead to delirium, the list of causes of dementias that can resemble AD dementia are relatively limited, and can be categorized into those that are reversible and those that are irreversible. This categorization serves 2 purposes. The first is that it emphasizes the importance to the diagnostician of first determining the presence of delirium; that is, dementia in the presence of a disturbance in consciousness. This step is not only important for the immediate care of the patient but is likely also to have long-term consequences, as delirium is the result of brain cells finding themselves in a toxic environment, whether the result of inflammation, electrolyte imbalance, inadequate oxygen or glucose supply, and so forth. Any extended period under these toxic conditions could potentially lead to irreversible consequences for patient's cognitive function in the future, regardless of successful eventual remediation of the toxic conditions. While the presence of delirium requires urgent corrective action, it also necessitates a subsequent investigation into the possibility of an underlying dementia. Both the aged brain and the demented brain have limited reserves that lead to increased susceptibility to developing delirium even under rather benign circumstances, such as a urinary tract infection. **Box 4** lists a set of tests suggested for an initial screening of patients presenting with delirium and/or dementia. **Box 5** lists the typical questions emphasized in a review of systems conducted with the patient and a knowledgable informant, the most significant aspects of the neurologic examination, and the brief bedside neuropsychological evaluation that in combination with the screening tests may be regarded as a template for an initial dementia evaluation.

In parallel to determining the presence of delirium, the diagnostician pursues reversible causes of dementia. Fortunately the reversible causes that are the most important not to miss are the easiest to rule out with laboratory tests. Potentially reversible causes include normal-pressure hydrocephalus vitamin deficiencies (eg,

---

Box 4
Frequently used screening tests for reversible causes of dementia and for delirium

Blood urea nitrogen, creatinine

Complete blood count

Electrolytes including magnesium

Electrocardiography

Erythrocyte sedimentation rate or C-reactive protein

Fasting glucose

Homocysteine

Lipid profile

Liver enzymes

Human immunodeficiency virus test, syphilis serology (eg, rapid plasma reagin)

Thyroid function tests

Urinalysis with microscopy

Vitamins: B_{12}, folate

Chest radiography

MR imaging or computed tomography scan (eliminate acute stroke, subdural hematoma, tumors)

Used Less Often:

Heavy metal screening and antinuclear antibodies

Lumbar puncture to obtain cerebrospinal fluid evaluation

Toxicology screens

Electroencephalography (seizures, Creutzfeldt-Jakob disease)

Ceruloplasmin, slit-lamp evaluation for Wilson disease

Titer for Lyme disease

Tests for Cushing and Conn diseases

---

vitamins B_1, B_6, B_{12}), endocrine diseases (eg, hypothyroidism, Cushing or Conn disease, diabetes), infectious diseases (syphilis, tuberculosis, Creutzfeldt-Jakob, fungal and viral), tumors, toxins, vasculitides (eg, lupus erythematosus, temporal arteritis), epilepsy, and psychiatric disorders (eg, major depressive) and sequelae of brain injury (eg, subdural hematoma). The irreversible causes are of neurodegenerative nature and are usually either secondary to cerebrovascular disease (eg, multiple infarct disease) or related to AD, as these all appear likely to some degree or another to feature an aggregating proteome (eg, frontotemporal disease and progressive supranuclear palsy). Laboratory tests are available for

---

Box 5
Examinations

Review of systems emphasizes questions related to:

Memory

Thinking

Forgetfulness

Disorientation

Misplacing objects, getting lost in familiar places, failure to recognize familiar people or objects

Difficulty performing everyday tasks such as peeling a potato or opening a can

Word-finding problems

Difficulty planning or organizing tasks (paying bills, cooking, housekeeping, driving, shopping)

Personality changes: irritability, motivation, depression

Neurologic examinations:

Presence of lateralizing signs

Signs of parkinsonism including gait and balance

Evidence of hyperreflexia

Test for frontal release and disinhibition

Tests for ideomotor apraxia

Test for ataxia

Brief neuropsychological evaluation:

Use of Mini Mental State Examination or Montreal Cognitive Assessment is common

Include tests of

Orientation

Attention

Calculations

Executive function (interpretation of proverbs, conceptualization)

Insight and judgment

Visuospatial abilities (clock drawing and copying of 2- and 3-dimensional figures)

Language (rate, rhythm, fluidity, latency, volume, grammar and syntax)

Writing and reading

Mood and affect

Phonemic and semantic fluency

Hallucinations and/or delusions

Ability to name all upper digits

---

most of the reversible causes. MR imaging and/or computed tomography perform well for discovery of tumor and cerebrovascular disease, and a variety of electroencephalographic measures for the determination of epilepsy are available. The diagnostician must then discriminate among the neurodegenerative diseases.

Although in general there is less clinical confusion about the presence of dementia, sometimes discriminating among the different irreversible neurodegenerative causes remains challenging. **Box 6** lists prototypical clinical presentations of the most common dementias that can be confused with AD. However, with an ever increasing number of sophisticated biological approaches being taken, there is reason to believe that we will see substantial improvements in our ability to discriminate among these dementias in the coming decade. These approaches are addressed only briefly here, as they are covered in more detail elsewhere in this issue. One of the guiding principles is that the first clinical manifestations of each of the dementias are dependent on those distributed networks most affected by the specific neuronal populations that are the first to be rendered dysfunctional or lost entirely. For example, when the frontal-striatal network is disrupted, attention and speed of processing are affected, with phonetic (letter) fluency generally more affected than semantic fluency, and cueing helps subjects on recall tasks; by contrast, when hippocampal networks are affected, as in AD, semantic fluency is more affected than phonetic fluency, and cueing is less effective on recall tasks. If there is sufficient neuronal loss then volumetric MR imaging reveals these locations, pointing toward a specific type of dementia, However, FDG PET and functional MR (fMR) imaging activation studies, or fMR imaging studies of resting networks are much more likely to pick up abnormalities in these networks earlier. This approach can only go so far, as we run into the same problems as occur when we discriminate among dementias based on clinical presentation, because the clinical symptoms are a reflection of the regions and networks affected. For example, some AD patients demonstrate early and disproportionately severe impairments in the frontal lobe resembling frontotemporal dementia. Genetics offers a potential alternative, but even mutations in the same genes can present with different phenotypes, presumably as the result of interactions with genetic variation in the rest of the genome and/or interactions with the environment. For example, mutations in MAPT (microtubule-associated protein tau), GRN (granulin), and C9ORF72 are prototypical genetic causes for frontotemporal dementia, yet some

Box 6
Clinical presentations of the most common dementias that can be confused with AD

Normal-Pressure Hydrocephalus (NPH)

Triad of dementia, incontinence, and gait disturbance; frequent psychiatric manifestations including depression and obsessive-compulsive disorder

Vascular Dementia (VD)

Fluctuating clinical picture with stepwise progression, decreased phonemic fluency, diminished focal deficits, multiple infarcts, early gait disturbance, diminished grammatical complexity of sentences

Frontotemporal Dementia (FTD)

Behavioral variant frontotemporal dementia (bvFTD). Onset usually between ages 45 and 65 years, second most common dementia in this age group; lethargy, apathy, lack of volitional acts, disinhibition with possible social and legal consequences; initially memory impairment is minimal and hallucinations and delusions relatively rare; overeating, particularly of sweets

Primary progressive aphasia (PPA). Speech and language are the first symptoms and may remain the only complaints for some time

Semantic dementia. Speech fluency is relatively intact, but patient loses the ability to understand the meaning of words and objects. Associated with ubiquitin or progranulin (TAR-DNA) mutation type, but occasionally AD

Progressive nonfluent aphasia. Speech requires considerable effort, and is nonfluent and agrammatic in nature, but patient retains ability to comprehend words. Evidence of a tau mutation, rarely AD

Logopenic progressive aphasia (LPA). Now considered to be an atypical form of AD. Patient exhibits deficits in naming and repetition in the context of intact syntax and motor speech. Logopenic is derived from the Greek "lack of words." Fluency is intermediate between fluent and nonfluent PPAs and less severe impairment with respect to semantic retrieval. Typically associated with AD

Some FTD patients may demonstrate motor neuron disease (amyotrophic lateral sclerosis)

Parkinson Disease Plus Dementias

Dementia with Lewy bodies (DLB). Recurrent fully formed visual hallucinations, parkinsonism, syncope, and repeated falls are common; systemized delusions, fluctuations in cognition and/or arousal, rapid eye movement (REM) sleep behavior disorder; initially attention, executive, and/or visuospatial functioning is most affected; usually hippocampal atrophy is minimal at onset and language usually not impaired; extreme sensitivity to neuroleptics, occipital hypoperfusion, and hypometabolism is frequent and slow-wave activity prominent on electroencephalogram

Parkinson disease with dementia (PDD). Initial motor signs preceding cognitive impairment by at least 12 months, but otherwise parallels DLB

Corticobasal syndrome (CBS). Sudden in onset and often asymmetric sensorimotor findings of akinesia, rigidity, apraxia (ideomotor and/or limb-kinetic), gait problems, possible numbness or needle-like sensation in limbs; may have difficulty initiating speech, alien hand syndrome (sensation may be late symptom)

Progressive supranuclear palsy (PSP). Seventh decade is usual age of onset with symmetric parkinsonism (gait disturbance, frequent falls, urinary incontinence, and constipation but usually no tremor); difficulty with eye movements including focusing on near objects and involuntary movements; may have personality changes; little or no response to L-DOPA

Multiple system atrophy (also known as Shy-Drager syndrome, striatonigral degeneration, and sporadic olivopontocerebellar atrophy). Rigidity, gait disturbance, difficulty initiating motor movements, little or no response to L-DOPA or dopaminergic agonists, autonomic dysfunction (incontinence or retention, impotence, hypotension); sleep problems may include REM behavior disorder and apnea; hypoperfusion and hypometabolism in cerebellum and striatum

individuals with these mutations appear clinically identical to those with AD and show AD postmortem pathology.[26] Ultimately, one will need to be able to assess the underlying initial causes of each dementia using biomarkers in the hope, of course, of using this knowledge not only to provide better diagnostic and prognostic information to patients, families, and caregivers, but also to provide an opportunity for early successful intervention.

REFERENCES

1. Alzheimer's Association. 2010 Alzheimer's disease facts and figures. Alzheimers Dement 2010;6: 158–94.
2. Galimberti D, Scarpini E. Progress in Alzheimer's disease. J Neurol 2012;259:201–11.
3. Hardy J, Selkoe DJ. The amyloid hypothesis of Alzheimer's disease: progress and problems on the road to therapeutics. Science 2002;297:353–6.
4. Zlokovic BV, Deane R, Sagare AP, et al. Low-density lipoprotein receptor-related protein-1: a serial clearance homeostatic mechanism controlling Alzheimer's amyloid β-peptide elimination from the brain. J Neurochem 2010;115:1077–89.
5. Cai Z, Zhao B, Ratka A. Oxidative stress and β-amyloid protein in Alzheimer's disease. Neuromolecular Med 2011;13:223–50.
6. Cummings JL, Doody R, Clark C. Disease modifying therapies for Alzheimer's disease. Neurology 2007; 69:1622–34.
7. Sparks DL, Scheff SW, Liu H, et al. Increased density of senile plaques (SP), but not neurofibrillary tangles (NFT), in non-demented individuals with the apolipoprotein E4 allele: comparison to confirmed Alzheimer's disease patients. J Neurol Sci 1996; 138(1–2):97–104.
8. Herrup K. Reimagining Alzheimer's disease—an age-based hypothesis. J Neurosci 2010;30(50): 16755–62.
9. David DC. Aging and the aggregating proteome. Front Genet 2012;3:247. http://dx.doi.org/10.3389/fgene.2012.00247.
10. Mancuso C, Scapagini G, Curro D, et al. Mitochondrial dysfunction, free radical generation and cellular stress response in neurodegenerative disorders. Front Biosci 2007;12:1107–23.
11. Lucin KM, Wyss-Coray T. Immune activation in brain aging and neurodegeneration: too much or too little. Neuron 2009;64:110–22.
12. Newington JT, Pitts A, Chien A, et al. Amyloid beta resistance in nerve cell lines is mediated by the Warburg effect. PLoS One 2011;6(4):e19191. http://dx.doi.org/10.1371/journal.pone.0019191.
13. Walker LC, Diamond MI, Duff KE, et al. Mechanisms of protein seeding in neurodegenerative diseases. JAMA Neurol 2013;70(3):304–10.
14. Eisele YS, Obemuller UO, Heilbronner G, et al. Peripherally applied Aβ-containing inoculates induce cerebral β-amyloidosis. Science 2010;330:980–2.
15. Braak H, Tredici KD. Alzheimer's pathogenesis: is there neuron-to-neuron propagation? Acta Neuropathol 2011;121:589–95.
16. Hollingworth P, Harold D, Jones L, et al. Alzheimer's disease genetics: current knowledge and future challenges. Int J Geriatr Psychiatry 2011;26:793–802.
17. Cruchaga C, Haller G, Chakraverty S, et al. Rare variants in APP, PSEN1 and PSEN2 increase risk for AD in late-onset Alzheimer's disease families. PLoS One 2012;7(2):e31039.
18. Wingo TS, Lah JJ, Levey AL, et al. Autosomal recessive causes likely in early-onset Alzheimer disease. Arch Neurol 2012;69:59.
19. Anstey KJ, Cherbuin N, Harath PM. Development of a new method for assessing global risk of Alzheimer's disease for use in population health approaches to prevention. Prev Sci 2013;14(4):411–21. http://dx.doi.org/10.1007/s11121-012-0313-2.
20. McGeer PL, Schulzer M, McGeer EG. Arthritis and anti-inflammatory agents as possible protective factors for Alzheimer's disease: a review of 17 epidemiologic studies. Neurology 1996;47:425–32.
21. Fillit H, Hess G, Hill J, et al. IV immunoglobulin is associated with a reduced risk of Alzheimer disease and related disorders. Neurology 2009;73: 180–5.
22. McKhann GM, Knopman DS, Chertkow H, et al. The diagnosis of dementia due to Alzheimer's disease: recommendations from the National Institute on Aging-Alzheimer's Association workgroups on diagnostic guidelines for Alzheimer's disease. Alzheimers Dement 2011;7:263–9.
23. Albert MS, DeKosky ST, Dickson D, et al. The diagnosis of mild cognitive impairment due to Alzheimer's disease: recommendations from the National Institute on Aging-Alzheimer's Association workgroups on diagnostic guidelines for Alzheimer's disease. Alzheimers Dement 2011;7(3):270–9.
24. Galton CJ, Patterson K, Xuereb JH, et al. Atypical and typical presentations of Alzheimer's disease: a clinical, neuropsychological, neuroimaging and pathological study of 13 cases. Brain 2000;123: 484–98.
25. Jack CR, Knopman DS, Weigand MS, et al. An operational approach to National Institute on Aging-Alzheimer's Association criteria for preclinical Alzheimer Disease. Ann Neurol 2012; 71(6):765–75.
26. Wojtas A, Heggeli KA, Finch N, et al. C9ORF72 repeat expansions and other FTD gene mutations in a clinical AD patient series from Mayo Clinic. Am J Neurodegener Dis 2012;1:107–18.

Structural and Functional Magnetic Resonance Imaging
Mild Cognitive Impairment and Alzheimer Disease

Hannah Lockau, MD[a], Frank Jessen, MD[b],
Andreas Fellgiebel, MD[c], Alexander Drzezga, MD[d],*

KEYWORDS

- Alzheimer disease • Dementia • Mild cognitive impairment • Magnetic resonance imaging
- Diffusion tensor imaging • Arterial spin labeling • Magnetic resonance spectroscopy

KEY POINTS

- The prevalence of clinically manifest Alzheimer disease (AD), representing a distinctly age-associated disorder, is growing in parallel with the increasing life expectancy in modern societies.
- It is well accepted today that the neuropathologic changes associated with AD develop in the brain years to decades ahead of the symptomatic onset, which limits the value of clinical assessment for early diagnosis.
- Structural imaging, namely magnetic resonance (MR) imaging, plays a pivotal role in the clinical management of dementia; this refers particularly to the exclusion of non-neurodegenerative causes of cognitive impairment, such as tumors, inflammation, or vascular abnormalities, and the assessment of regional brain atrophy.
- The introduction of advanced instrumentation such as 7-T MR imaging, as well as new or improved MR imaging sequences such as arterial spin labeling, MR spectroscopy, diffusion tensor imaging, and resting-state functional MR imaging, may open new pathways toward the improved diagnosis of AD, even in early stages of disease such as mild cognitive impairment.

INTRODUCTION

Alzheimer disease (AD) represents a strongly age-associated disorder, showing an almost exponential increase with age.[1] More than 20% of persons older than 80 years are affected by clinically manifest dementia.[2,3] Because of increasing life expectancy, the prevalence of this fatal disorder is continuously rising, already reaching more than 5 million people in the United States today.[3] In many countries the elderly population is growing disproportionately. For example, in the United

Disclosures: This work was supported by grants of the German Research Foundation (DFG) DR 445/4-1 to Alexander Drzezga. Alexander Drzezga has worked as a consultant for Bayer Healthcare, Siemens Healthcare, GE Healthcare, Piramal, Avid/Lilly Pharmaceuticals. Andreas Fellgiebel acts as a consultant for GE Healthcare and Avid/Lilly Pharmaceuticals. Frank Jessen received consultation fees and speakers honoraria from GE Healthcare, Lilly, Novartis, Esai, Pfizer, Jansen-Cilag, Schwabe and Nutricia.

[a] Department of Radiology, University Hospital Cologne, Kerpener Street 62, Cologne 50937, Germany; [b] Department of Psychiatry, German Center for Neurodegenerative Diseases (DZNE), University of Bonn, Sigmund-Freud-Straße 25, Bonn 53105, Germany; [c] Department of Psychiatry and Psychotherapy, University Medical Center Mainz, Untere Zahlbacher Street 8, Mainz 55131, Germany; [d] Department of Nuclear Medicine, University Hospital Cologne, Kerpener Street 62, Cologne 50937, Germany
* Corresponding author.
E-mail address: alexander.drzezga@uk-koeln.de

PET Clin 8 (2013) 407–430
http://dx.doi.org/10.1016/j.cpet.2013.08.004
1556-8598/13/$ – see front matter © 2013 Elsevier Inc. All rights reserved.

States the number of persons aged 65 years and older is projected to double by 2030, and thus the incidence of AD is expected to approach nearly a million new patients per year.[4] Consequently, this disorder will represent an enormous burden in the future not only for the patients and their relatives but also with regard to the socioeconomic system. It is well accepted today that the neuropathology underlying AD starts years to decades before the onset of clinical symptoms.[5,6] Subjects may then go through a phase of subjective cognitive complaints, followed by a stage of mild cognitive impairment (MCI), which is characterized by objective measurable deficits in cognitive performance, not yet sufficient for a diagnosis of dementia.[7] Finally, the stage of clinically manifest dementia is characterized by cognitive problems severe enough to impair the capabilities of daily living.[8,9]

This insidious progress of the disease implicates that millions of people are living among us with Alzheimer-type neuropathology already developing in their brain, without being diagnosed or even showing any symptoms. Traditionally, the clinical diagnosis of AD according to corresponding guidelines required the proof of manifest dementia based on the symptomatic appearance, including (1) confirmation of cognitive impairment affecting activities of daily living by means of neuropsychological assessment and interviews with the patient and informants (eg, spouse or children), and (2) the exclusion of causes other than AD for the cognitive decline.[9] Biomarkers played a subordinate role in this diagnostic approach, and imaging has only been recommended to exclude non-neurodegenerative reasons for cognitive impairment such as inflammation, tumors, or vascular problems. Obviously such a strategy would not allow identification of patients in early stages of disease, given that clinically manifest dementia represents a late stage of AD from a neuropathologic perspective.

Regarding this shortcoming, the new diagnostic entity MCI (mild cognitive impairment) has been introduced in recent years. The diagnosis of MCI requires objective cognitive impairment in comparison with age-matched healthy subjects, which, however, does not yet affect the activities of daily living. The group of patients with MCI can be regarded as a population at risk for development of AD-type dementia, because a relatively high percentage (15%–30%) of these patients will progress to manifest dementia within a short period of time. However, the MCI group is very heterogeneous and contains patients with other neuropsychiatric disorders (eg, depression), so their cognitive symptoms may remain stable or

even improve over time.[7] Based on clinical assessment, a reliable prognosis cannot therefore be established during the stage of MCI.

For many years treatment options of AD have been mainly symptomatic (eg, acetylcholine esterase inhibitors), thus the diagnosis of AD ahead of the symptomatic stage may have appeared of little value. In recent years, however, huge efforts have been made to develop causal therapy strategies. Most of these efforts are mainly directed toward the reduction of β-amyloid aggregation pathology in the brain, which includes the secretase blockers and vaccination strategies.[10] Thus far, however, no therapeutic breakthrough has been achieved with these new treatment approaches. It has been proposed that it may be crucial to start with any causal therapy for AD during mildly or even asymptomatic stages, that is, before irreversible neuronal damage. Thus the need for reliable and sensitive disease biomarkers has become more obvious. Furthermore, the relatively slow progression of the disease as well as the limited correlation between the severity of cognitive symptoms and the extent of neuropathology in the brain underline the need for diagnostic tools that are suitable for the monitoring of quantitative therapy.

These considerations may have fostered the trend in Europe and the United States to include biomarkers in current guidelines and research criteria for the diagnosis of dementia of the Alzheimer type, for MCI due to AD and even for probable AD in preclinical stages.[11-14] In brief, these criteria include cerebrospinal fluid (CSF) markers but also imaging tools such as amyloid imaging and imaging of glucose metabolism (^{18}F-fluorodeoxyglucose [FDG]) with PET as well as structural MR imaging. Positivity for amyloid in PET or CSF is regarded as an early finding predisposing for the development of AD, whereas abnormalities observed with FDG PET or structural MR imaging are considered markers of neuronal loss (ie, reflecting the onset of manifest neurodegeneration). A combination of amyloid positivity and neuronal loss is considered a strong indicator for the presence of AD pathology. This categorization may represent an oversimplification to some extent, given the fact that FDG PET rather allows the measurement of neuronal dysfunction, which may occur ahead of manifest neuronal loss as measured with MR imaging. Indeed many studies were able to demonstrate a higher sensitivity of FDG PET compared with structural MR imaging with regard, for example, to prognosis in MCI.[15] However, FDG PET may not be broadly available and even when it is accessible, structural MR imaging is always recommended for exclusion of non-neurodegenerative causes of cognitive impairment. Thus, a profound knowledge about typical findings in structural MR imaging associated with different stages of AD and other forms of neurodegeneration represents an essential part of the armamentarium of any imaging expert active in this field.

In addition to the well-established clinical MR imaging procedures, advanced instrumentation such as 7-T MR imaging, as well as of new or improved MR imaging sequences such as arterial spin labeling (ASL), MR spectroscopy, diffusion tensor (DT) imaging, and resting-state functional MR (fMR) imaging are finding their way into the assessment of neurodegenerative disorders. These developments may open new pathways toward improved diagnosis and functional assessment of AD even in the early stages of disease such as MCI. The purpose of this article is to describe the typical findings of established as well as of newer MR imaging procedures in healthy aging, MCI, and AD.

MR IMAGING–BASED EXCLUSION OF NON-NEURODEGENERATIVE CAUSES OF COGNITIVE IMPAIRMENT

At initial presentation, a thorough clinical examination and survey of the patient's history is mandatory in the dementia workup. Patients and relatives should be formally interviewed about the onset and duration of symptoms, if the disease is rapidly progressive, and if clinical risk factors for non-neurodegenerative reasons of cognitive decline such as vascular disorders, history of neoplasm, infection, inflammation, or trauma are known.[16] Even if these risk factors can be excluded, structural imaging of the brain is crucial in demented patients for exclusion of underlying cerebral disease other than neurodegeneration and with regard to prognosis and further treatment. Differential diagnoses are numerous and cannot be discussed here in detail, thus only some major aspects are highlighted. Compared with computed tomography (CT), MR imaging provides the advantage of a higher contrast of soft tissue in general, and of gray and white matter in particular. Therefore, it is regarded as the imaging method of choice for patients with symptoms of central nervous system (CNS) disorders.

T2-weighted and/or fluid-attenuated inversion recovery (FLAIR)-weighted images are sensitive for the detection of white matter damage resulting in gliosis or focal edema, which usually accompanies any parenchymal abnormality. Leukoencephalopathy, with or without additional lacunar or territorial parenchymal defects, is a typical finding

in patients with vascular dementia. Any neoplastic, metabolic, or inflammatory disease presents with focal or diffuse edema, which is best detected as hyperintensity on T2-weighted/FLAIR images.

Idiopathic normal-pressure hydrocephalus (NPH) is an important (and usually treatable) differential diagnosis in patients with the classic clinical triad of dementia, gait apraxia, and urinary incontinence. The typical MR imaging findings are a symmetric dilatation of the ventricles and the Sylvian fissures out of proportion to sulcal enlargement, and without atrophy of the hippocampus. Periventricular FLAIR/T2-weighted hyperintensity represents transependymal CSF flow (**Fig. 1**, **Table 1**).

Gradient echo T2*-weighted images are mandatory for the detection of hematoma or microbleeds, which can be an accidental finding in the aging brain, but can also be found in patients with cerebral amyloid angiopathy (CAA) or hypertensive encephalopathy. In CAA, microbleeds are typically distributed in cortical/subcortical regions with emphasis on the frontomesial, fronto-orbital, and parietal regions.[17] Involvement of the basal ganglia is rare in amyloid angiopathy and is suggestive of causative arteriolosclerosis.[18] It is essential to detect vascular disease of the brain parenchyma, because vascular dementia may represent a relatively frequent differential diagnosis of neurodegenerative dementias. However, it is commonly accepted today that there is a major overlap between typical pathology of AD and vascular dementia. Thus, the proof of vascular abnormality does not exclude the coexistence of a neurodegenerative disorder, and vice versa. Nevertheless, the detection of vascular abnormalities is crucial, as they may represent potentially treatable cofactors (eg, hypertension) with an influence on the overall prognosis of AD and other forms of dementia.

For imaging criteria and an example of subcortical arteriosclerotic encephalopathy (hypertensive encephalopathy), see **Table 1** and **Fig. 2**.

Diffusion-weighted (DW) imaging should also be part of a standard protocol for dementia to exclude acute ischemic infarction and to help identify patients suffering from infectious diseases such as herpes encephalitis (**Fig. 3**; see **Table 1**) or prion disease. Creutzfeldt-Jakob disease (CJD) and its variants show typical MR imaging findings with high diagnostic sensitivity, attributable to a specific pattern with hyperintense lesions within the basal ganglia on DW, T2-weighted, and FLAIR-weighted images.[19] An important differential diagnosis to herpes encephalitis as a cause of rapidly progressive dementias is limbic encephalitis (**Fig. 4**). Limbic encephalitis as an autoimmune inflammatory disease of the brain is paraneoplastic

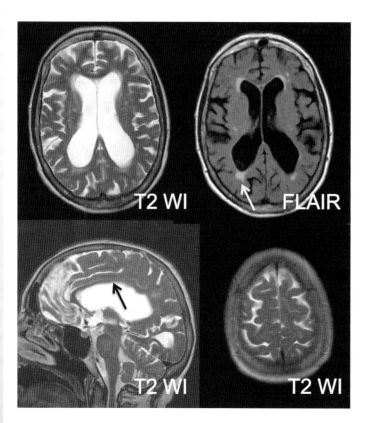

Fig. 1. Normal-pressure hydrocephalus. Symmetrically dilated ventricles, disproportional to sulcal enlargement (T2-weighted image [T2 WI]). Fluid-attenuated inversion recovery (FLAIR) hyperintense periventricular signal caused by transependymal cerebrospinal fluid flow (*white arrow*). Bowing and thinning of corpus callosum (*black arrow*).

in most cases and, as the name suggests, primarily affects the limbic structures. Differential diagnosis to herpes encephalitis based on MR imaging alone can be difficult or even impossible, as imaging findings are very similar. T2-weighted/FLAIR hyperintensity of the affected structures, diffusion restriction, and subtle mass effect as well as patchy contrast enhancement can be found in both entities. Microbleeds in later stages of the disease can confound the diagnosis of herpes encephalitis,[20,21] as these findings are absent in limbic encephalitis.

Another inflammatory autoimmune disease to bear in mind concerning the differential diagnosis of cognitive impairment is multiple sclerosis (MS). History of focal neurologic deficits especially in young to middle-aged woman should raise suspicion. Typical imaging findings are multiple supratentorial T2-weighted/FLAIR-hyperintense ovoid lesions with a mainly periventricular location and involvement of the corpus callosum. Presence of subcortical and infratentorial lesions as well as contrast enhancement and/or diffusion restriction in active inflammation help to confirm the diagnosis. In later stages of the disease, diffuse brain atrophy can be found.[22–24]

Changes in brain tissue as a consequence of some metabolic/toxic diseases such as Wernicke encephalopathy, with its typical imaging pattern of T2-weighted/FLAIR hyperintensity in periaqueductal gray matter and around the third ventricle can also show restricted diffusion (**Fig. 5**; see **Table 1**).

Contrast-enhanced T1 weighted images are helpful for further evaluation if the T2-weighted/FLAIR images point to brain neoplasm such as CNS lymphoma (**Fig. 6**; see **Table 1**) or meningeal/parenchymal infection, as well as inflammation. In all cases of rapidly progressive dementia, contrast-enhanced sequences should be mandatory. **Table 2** and **Fig. 7** show an example of an imaging protocol.

MR IMAGING METHODS FOR SPECIFIC ASSESSMENT OF NEURODEGENERATIVE CHANGES

In daily clinical routine, radiologic assessment of dementia patients is mainly based on standard structural MR imaging protocols acquired on scanners with field strengths of 1.5 or 3 T. Advanced scanning techniques, such as the installation of the first 7-T scanners for humans at certain research sites, may provide additional information.

Table 1
Examples of differential diagnoses of non-neurodegenerative dementing diseases showing main imaging findings and sequences

Etiology	Diagnosis	Diagnostic Clues
Vascular	Subcortical arteriosclerotic encephalopathy (see **Fig. 2**)	General findings: confluent supratentorial periventricular WMLs and lacunar defects with involvement of basal ganglia and brainstem, microbleeds with involvement of basal ganglia T2 WI/FLAIR: Confluent ↑ WMLs, lacunae T2*: microbleeds, basal ganglia involved
Infectious	Herpes encephalitis (see **Fig. 3**)	General findings: affection of limbic system, medial temporal lobe, inferior frontal lobe common. Bilateral but often asymmetric, subtle mass effect T2 WI/FLAIR: ↑ cortical/subcortical signal of affected structures DWI: diffusion restriction usually present, may be early sign T1 WI CE: patchy to gyriform enhancement T2*: microhemorrhages possible
Neoplastic	(Primary) CNS lymphoma (see **Fig. 6**)	General findings: Local mass, supratentorial periventricular location common, corpus callosum and basal ganglia can be involved, solitary/multiple lesions T2 WI/FLAIR: ↓/isointense to cortex, hyperintense perifocal edema T1 WI CE: Enhancement homogeneous or peripheral DWI: May show diffusion restriction Noncontrast CT: hyperdense
Paraneoplastic	Limbic encephalitis (see **Fig. 4**)	General findings: mimics herpes encephalitis! T2 WI/FLAIR: ↑ signal in medial temporal lobes and limbic system, subtle mass effect possible T1 WI CE: patchy/gyriform enhancement T2*: no hemorrhage (DD herpes encephalitis) DWI: Shows diffusion restriction
Metabolic/toxic	Wernicke encephalopathy (see **Fig. 5**)	General findings: Signal changes in periaqueductal gray matter, around third ventricle, mammillary bodies. Normal MR image ≠ exclusion of Wernicke encephalopathy! T2 WI/FLAIR: ↑ signal of affected structures T1 WI CE: can show enhancement
Others	Normal-pressure hydrocephalus (see **Fig. 1**)	General findings: symmetrically dilated ventricles, dilated Sylvian fissure (disproportional to general sulcal enlargement, fourth ventricle relatively spared) T2 WI/FLAIR: ↑ periventricular signal (transependymal CSF flow) Sagittal T1 WI/T2 WI: bowing/thinning of corpus callosum (CSF flow study: increase of flow in aqueduct)

Abbreviations: ↑, hyperintense; ↓, hypointense; CE, contrast enhanced; CNS, central nervous system; CSF, cerebrospinal fluid; CT, computed tomography; DD, differential diagnosis; DWI, diffusion-weighted imaging; FLAIR, fluid-attenuated inversion recovery; WI, weighted imaging; WML, white matter lesion.

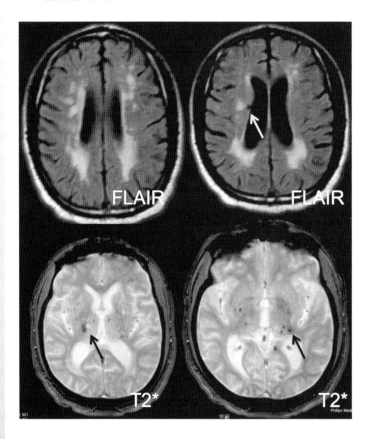

Fig. 2. Subcortical arteriosclerotic leukoencephalopathy. FLAIR hyperintense white matter lesions, lacunar parenchymal defects possible (*white arrow*). Microbleeds in T2*-weighted imaging with involvement of basal ganglia (*black arrow*).

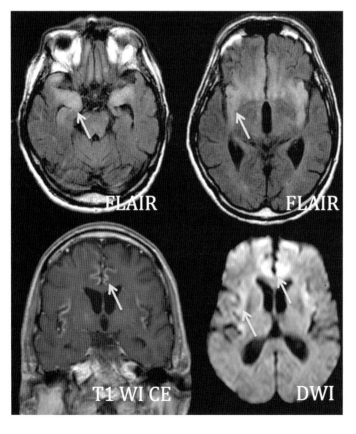

Fig. 3. Herpes encephalitis. Limbic structures with hyperintense signal in FLAIR-weighted images (note subtle mass effect), diffusion restriction (diffusion-weighted [DWI]), and gyriform/patchy contrast enhancement (T1-weighted contrast enhanced [T1 WI CE]) (*white arrows* indicate major imaging findings).

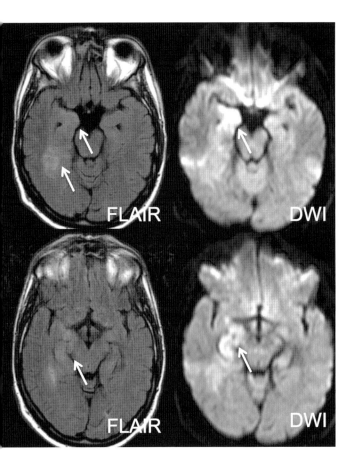

Fig. 4. Limbic encephalitis. FLAIR hyperintensity and restricted diffusion (DWI) of limbic structures (*white arrows*).

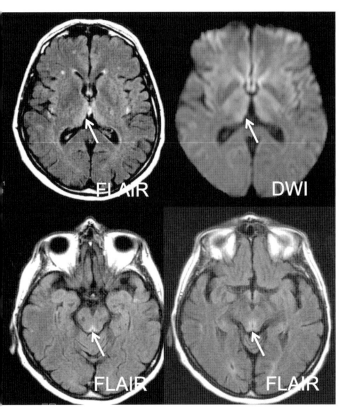

Fig. 5. Wernicke encephalopathy. High signal in periaqueductal gray matter and around third ventricle (*white arrows*) on FLAIR-weighted images. Note subtle diffusion restriction (DWI).

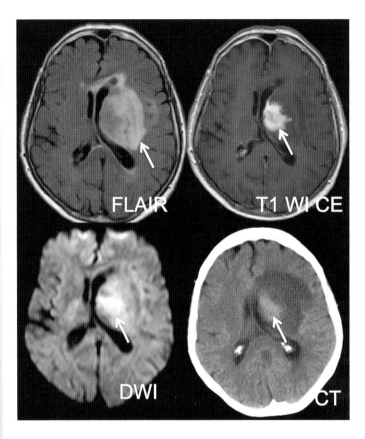

Fig. 6. Primary CNS lymphoma: Periventricular supratentorial mass with homogeneous contrast enhancement (T1 WI CE), restricted diffusion (DWI), and FLAIR hyperintense perifocal edema. Hyperdensity in non–contrast-enhanced CT scan is typical (*white arrows* indicate major imaging findings).

Oblique coronal image acquisition is useful for the assessment of the hippocampal region. The precise definition of the hippocampal volume is an important diagnostic tool in defining AD atrophy patterns. To date the most accurate way of volumetry is by manual definition of hippocampal borders in a rather time-consuming procedure.[25]

Voxel-based morphometry is widely used in dementia research studies for voxelwise comparison of the percentage amount of gray matter between

Table 2
Example of a clinical imaging protocol for assessment of dementia

Dimension	Sequence	Major Information
3D or oblique coronal 2D	3 mm or 3D T1 WI	Evaluate medial temporal lobe/hippocampal region in aspects of atrophy
Axial	4 mm FLAIR and 4 mm T2 WI	White matter pathology (eg, due to infection, vascular disorders, neoplasm), parenchymal defects, atrophy pattern in T2 WI
Axial	4 mm T2* WI	Hemorrhage, microbleeds (eg, arteriolosclerosis, cerebral amyloid angiopathy)
Axial and if possible coronal/sagittal	4 mm DWI	Infarction, inflammation/infection (eg, prion disease, herpes encephalitis), coronal/sagittal DWI can be helpful for assessment of brainstem
Axial and if possible coronal/sagittal	Contrast- enhanced 4 mm T1 WI	Further evaluation (eg, infection, brain tumor). Should be applied in rapidly progressive dementias

Abbreviations: 2D, 2-dimensional; 3D, 3-dimensional; DWI, diffusion-weighted imaging; FLAIR, fluid-attenuated inversion recovery; WI, weighted imaging.

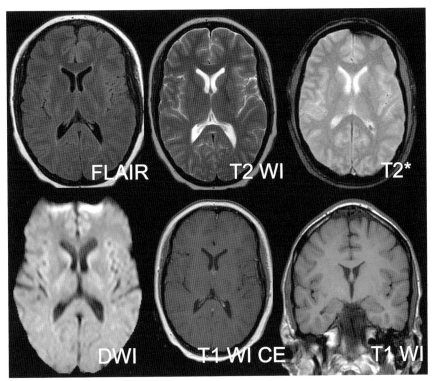

Fig. 7. Standard MR imaging sequences in a healthy subject as an example for a typical imaging protocol. DWI, diffusion-weighted image; FLAIR, fluid-attenuated inversion recovery; T1 WI CE, T1-weighted contrast-enhanced image.

2 groups of subjects or in 1 patient versus a group of control subjects. Following spatial normalization and segmentation of the gray matter, statistical tests for voxelwise comparison of the 2 groups are performed.[26]

Automated measurement methods for the assessment of the cortical thickness are another tool in the diagnostic armamentarium of AD in structural imaging, and have been developed and used in several studies during the past years.[27–29]

However, the adoption of these techniques into the routine clinical setting is not applicable, and therefore the diagnosis of hippocampal volume loss is usually made on the visual aspect on coronal T1-weighted images in combination with transverse T2-weighted images. Visual rating scales (eg, Scheltens scale and Pasquier scale) have been developed to provide a practical tool for the graduation of cortical and hippocampal atrophy in clinical radiology.[30–32]

However, loss of brain volume has been demonstrated in different forms of neurodegeneration and also in healthy aging, which limits the diagnostic value of volumetric assessment of MR imaging data. Functional/molecular imaging procedures such as single-photon emission CT and PET may complement the MR imaging–based methods, particularly with reference to the well-established measurement of cerebral glucose metabolism by means of FDG PET, which has proved to be highly valuable for early diagnosis of AD even in the stage of MCI, and for the differential diagnosis between different forms of dementia.[33–36] Recently, PET tracers to detect cerebral amyloid deposits have been introduced, which may be suitable for the detection of AD pathology even in the very early (asymptomatic) stages, and with the goal of enrolling patients into new antiamyloid therapy trials.[37]

Corresponding modern MR imaging procedures to evaluate brain function, brain perfusion and brain metabolism are currently still a matter of research. In the future, these techniques may contribute to a better understanding of the pathophysiology of AD and therefore might help to predict the clinical course of the disease. Moreover, MR techniques may allow the identification of healthy individuals who are at an increased risk for AD.[38]

ASL is an imaging method that provides quantitative information about brain perfusion. The principle of this technique is the labeling of protons in arterial blood proximally to the field of image acquisition by an inversion pulse that will then function as an endogenous, freely diffusible tracer.[39] Repetitive scans of the same slice with and without prior labeling are made to optimize differentiation between signal of blood bolus and noise. This procedure is totally noninvasive, as no contrast agents have to be applied.

DT imaging is based on Brownian molecular motion of water molecules in the brain, with acquisition of diffusion of molecules in all 3 dimensions. The molecular diffusion within the white matter (other than, eg, the diffusion in the CSF) is restricted by different intercellular and intracellular structures, resulting in directionally dependent (anisotropic) motion along axonal bundles. By using 6 or more gradients, anisotropy (direction of diffusion) can be quantified by means of a voxel-by-voxel technique.[40] DT imaging provides evidence about regional density and integrity of axonal bundles, because diffusivity correlates with axonal density.[41]

[1]H MR spectroscopy provides a noninvasive technique for quantitative measurement of distinct brain metabolites in vivo. Similar to conventional/structural MR imaging, MR spectroscopy is mainly based on the proton signal. However, in principle other metabolites can also be used for MR spectroscopy.

In MR spectroscopy of the normal brain, N-acetylaspartate combined with N-acetylaspartylglutamate, a marker for neuronal integrity that is present in neuronal cells of gray matter as well as in axons, has the highest peak (in parts per million). A high choline peak (Cho, constituent of choline, phosphorylocholine, and glycerophosphorylcholine) is significant for highly proliferative tissue. The third important metabolite that is routinely evaluated in MR spectroscopy is creatine (Cr), a metabolite in aerobic glycolysis. Myo-inositol, a sugar-like precursor molecule of membrane phospholipids and phosphoinositides, is mainly located in glial cells.[42] In MR spectroscopy, therefore, myo-inositol is considered to be a glial marker. With regard to AD research, myo-inositol is considered to be an important metabolite associated with inflammatory changes.

The electrophysiologic basis of fMR imaging is the linkage between activation of brain areas during execution of cognitive tasks and brain perfusion. The most widely used fMR imaging technique is based on the so-called BOLD effect (blood oxygenation level dependent). An increase in cell metabolism caused by neuronal activation requires an increase in oxygen supply. To ensure this regional brain perfusion, it is adjusted by autoregulative mechanisms known as hemodynamic response. An increased supply of oxygenated hemoglobin due to increased perfusion is usually greater than necessary, thus resulting in increased washout of deoxygenated hemoglobin. The oxyhemoglobin/deoxyhemoglobin ratio therefore shifts from paramagnetic deoxyhemoglobin toward diamagnetic oxyhemoglobin, which leads to subtle changes in the $T2^*$ signal.

In contrast to fMR imaging activation studies, resting-state fMR imaging represents a method based on the acquisition of the BOLD signal in the absence of any cognitive task/interaction of the subject with the environment. The obtained information on spontaneous brain activity of the "resting" brain can be used to detect brain regions that exhibit strong correlations in their fluctuations of activity over time. These brain regions are considered to communicate to each other, that is, to be functionally connected. Studies using this method have led to the identification of several networks of functional connectivity, the most prominent being the so-called default network.[43–45] Disruption of the default network with changes in the functional connectivity of involved brain regions has been found in several brain diseases such as AD, schizophrenia, and autism.[46–50]

STRUCTURAL IMAGING

Any individual's brain is affected by aging processes. Differentiation of changes that are within the physiologic range of normal aging from pathologic findings represents one of the major challenges for MR imaging in elderly patients. Common observations in the aging brain include a certain degree of volume loss with subsequent enlargement of the perivascular spaces and CSF spaces, as well as unspecific hyperintense changes of the white matter or scattered microbleeds.[51–54] In the normal aging brain, atrophy rates of hippocampus at around 1% per year have been described.[55]

As mentioned earlier, MCI represents a risk condition for the development of AD, and in progressive patients can be considered a transitional cognitive state between healthy aging and dementia.[7] Rates of progression to AD have been reported in 10% to 15% of patients with MCI per year.[56,57] Structural MR imaging evaluating atrophy of the hippocampus has been shown to be able to predict later conversion to AD in up to 80% of MCI patients.[58,59] Apart from the hippocampus, the entorhinal cortex (ERC) has been discussed as a second brain region to show early alterations in volume. Volumetry of the ERC may therefore contribute to early diagnosis as an additional target.[60,61] Studies using voxel-based morphometry in MCI patients showed involvement

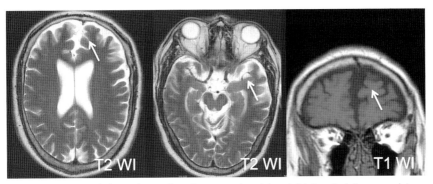

Fig. 8. Pronounced asymmetric bilateral atrophy of temporal and frontal lobes (*white arrows*) in a patient with suspected diagnosis of frontotemporal dementia.

of the mesiotemporal lobe and lateral association areas of the temporal and parietal lobes.[60,62,63]

With progression from MCI to AD, thinning of the entire cortex, especially in the temporal lobes, with pronouncement of the left hemisphere has been shown.[64] A study by Querbes and colleagues[27] showed that conversion from MCI to AD could be accurately predicted using an automated method of cortical-thickness measurement, with a predictive value of 76%.

It has been demonstrated that the rate of atrophy in MCI may be able to even more accurately predict conversion to AD.[65–67] However, the repetitive imaging approach required for longitudinal assessment is not well suited as a clinical test for everyday clinical routine.

In AD patients, again the temporal lobe, and especially the hippocampus and entorhinal cortex, is predominantly affected by atrophy.[68,69] Visual rating (eg, Scheltens scale) of medial temporal atrophy with evaluation of hippocampal volume, width of choroid fissure, and width of the temporal horn has been shown to hold diagnostic value.[70] However, atrophy of these structures is not specific for Alzheimer dementia. Marked temporal atrophy can also be found, for example, in frontotemporal dementia (FTD). FTD is a neurodegenerative disorder belonging to the group of frontotemporal lobar degenerative disorders (FTLD). FTLD summarizes several clinical syndromes, namely FTD, the progressive aphasias, and semantic dementia (sometimes referred to as semantic variant of progressive aphasia). Clinical symptoms, pathology, and genetics of these disorders are heterogenous.[71] However, as suggested by the name, atrophy of the temporal and/or frontal lobes is commonly observed in FTLD syndromes,[72] but pronouncement of atrophy varies between subtypes (**Fig. 8**). As an example, primary progressive aphasia (PPA), one of the subtypes of FTLD named by the leading clinical symptom of aphasia, presents with an imaging pattern of asymmetric temporal atrophy that is usually accentuated on the left hemisphere.[73] **Fig. 9** shows an imaging example of a patient with a suspected diagnosis of PPA at an early stage of the disease.

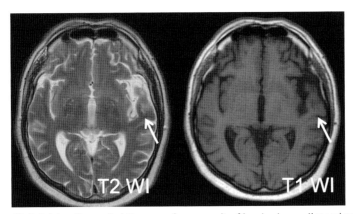

Fig. 9. Enlargement of left Sylvian fissure (*white arrows*) as a result of beginning unilateral temporal atrophy in a patient with suspected diagnosis of primary progressive aphasia.

In dementia with Lewy bodies (DLB), another example of a neurodegenerative disorder, the medial temporal lobe is relatively preserved in comparison with AD.[74] General brain atrophy is found in most patients with DLB, but pronounced temporal atrophy makes other neurodegenerative diseases such as AD or FTD more likely than DLB, and therefore can contribute to the diagnostic decision.

Regarding longitudinal assessment, hippocampal atrophy with percentual loss of up to 7% of the volume per year has been reported in AD.[75,76] Thus, particularly with regard to longitudinal assessment (eg, for therapy monitoring), volumetry and visual rating of hippocampal atrophy may serve as a diagnostic biomarker for disease progression of AD, even in a clinical setting (**Fig. 10**).

Whole-brain atrophy and degree of ventricular expansion over time are also percentually higher in AD patients than in cognitive normal elderly subjects. As reviewed by Frisoni and colleagues,[77] the ventricles of AD patients have been demonstrated to expand by 5% to 16% per year, compared with 1.5% to 3% in the normal aging population.

Reduction of cortical gray matter detected by voxel-based morphometry is present in the medial and lateral temporal lobe as well as in parietal association areas.[78,79] In some studies, measurement of the thickness of the temporal, orbitofrontal, and parietal cortex has been found to provide 90% to 100% sensitivity for differentiation of AD patients from healthy controls (**Fig. 11**).[28,29] Regarding the fact that medial temporal atrophy can also occur in frontotemporal lobar degeneration,[80,81] parietal cortical atrophy in addition to temporal atrophy may help to differentiate AD from other neurodegenerative diseases.[77] In summary, atrophy is a consistent finding in neurodegenerative disorders and particularly in AD, and visual rating of cortical and hippocampal atrophy can be practically applied as a diagnostic biomarker for the clinical evaluation of patients assessed for neurodegenerative disorders.

However, the fact that loss of brain volume is also present in other neurodegenerative disorders and is a physiologic phenomenon, even in healthy aging, limits its diagnostic value. Thus in the

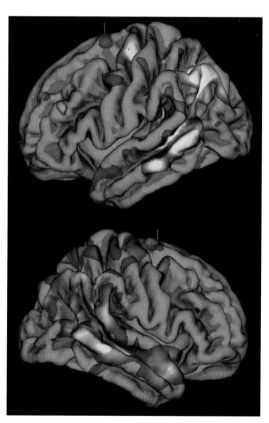

Fig. 11. Cortical thickness analysis in a group of patients with AD in comparison with healthy controls. Regions with significantly reduced cortical thickness in patients with AD are displayed in blue on a standard MR imaging template (left lateral and right lateral aspects of the brain) at a significance threshold of *P*<.01. (*Courtesy of* Freesurfer, Athinoula A. Martinos Center for Biomedical Imaging; and Peter Bohn, Munich, Germany.)

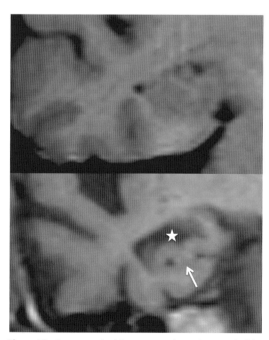

Fig. 10. Decreased hippocampal volume (*white arrow*) and enlargement of temporal horn (*asterisk*) in an AD patient (*bottom*). For comparison, a coronal T1-weighted image of the temporal lobe of a healthy middle-aged person is displayed (*top*).

guidelines of the American Academy of Neurology, MR imaging volumetry is not recommended as a valuable clinical tool for dementia assessment. In these guidelines it is proposed that the range of estimates suggests that measurement of hippocampal atrophy by MR imaging may not be useful in clinical practice because of its low precision. The investigators mention that FDG PET appears superior to MR imaging measures of hippocampal atrophy, because changes in cerebral glucose metabolism antedate the onset of memory decline whereas the hippocampal changes on MR imaging do not.[82] Correspondingly, a large meta-analysis demonstrated that FDG PET is superior to structural MR imaging with regard to prediction of AD at the stage of MCI.[15] On the other hand, more recent recommendations from the National Institute on Aging Alzheimer's Association work groups on diagnostic guidelines for AD suggest that structural MR imaging may be used as a marker of neuronal injury even in early preclinical stages of AD and in MCI. However, also in these recommendations, biomarkers of amyloid deposition (eg, PET amyloid imaging) are suggested to capture the onset of AD-typical pathology earlier in comparison with structural abnormalities.[11–13]

White matter lesions (WMLs) and microbleeds are incidental findings in the aging brain independent of Alzheimer dementia.[51] However, most studies on distribution and frequency of WMLs showed an increased lesion load in subcortical and periventricular areas in AD patients when compared with healthy controls.[83–86] A higher frequency of microbleeds in AD patients has also been reported, with predominance of occipital cortical/subcortical location.[87] White matter changes tend to progress over time, with higher progression rates in AD patients and can be associated with a rapid cognitive decline.[88] A high prevalence of microbleeds has been described in AD patients relative to the general population, and an association with a poor cognitive performance has been proposed.[87,89–92] As mentioned earlier, the potential to treat factors underlying cerebrovascular abnormalities (eg, hypertension) justifies the importance of detecting microbleeds and WMLs on clinical MR scans of patients suspected for AD. The amount of white matter hyperintensities on T2/FLAIR-weighted images can be estimated using a visual scale introduced by Fazekas and colleagues[52] on a 4-point scale from 0 to 3 (0 = absence of deep white matter hyperintense signals, 1 = punctuate foci, 2 = beginning confluence of foci, 3 = large confluent areas).

For an overview of the main aspects of image interpretation in a clinical setting, see **Box 1**.

Box 1
Important aspects to focus on while assessing MR imaging in a possible AD patient

Interpretative pearls and pitfalls for assessment of clinical MR imaging scans in Alzheimer dementia

Pearls:

Note decrease of gyral size, increase of sulcal size; Pasquier scale can be helpful[31,32]

Note accentuation of temporal and parietal lobe

Enlarged ventricles with temporal accentuation?

In coronal T1-weighted images visually assess volume of medial temporal lobe, focus on hippocampus and entorhinal cortex; Scheltens scale can be helpful[30]

Presence of white matter changes and microbleeds?

White matter changes show higher progression rates in AD (cognitive decline can be associated); Fazekas scale can be helpful[52,88]

Progression on repeated scans if available?

Pitfalls:

Findings suggestive of other dementing diseases?

Temporal atrophy in other neurodegenerative dementias (eg, frontotemporal dementia)

DIFFUSION TENSOR IMAGING

The application of DT imaging (**Fig. 12**) to the quantitative study of the effects of normal aging has provided new insights into age-related and functionally relevant changes of white matter microstructure. Using DT imaging, distinct patterns of white matter and hippocampal alterations have also been reported in MCI and AD. In AD different white matter abnormalities including decreased myelin density, loss of oligodendrocytes, and microglial activation have been reported.[93–95] Of note, the loss of oligodendrocytes and myelin damage in AD has been postulated to occur because of increased vulnerability of later myelinating regions.[96–98] Moreover, frequent microvascular changes in AD[99] and Wallerian degeneration of fiber connections resulting from cortical neuronal loss are likely to contribute to the white matter changes in AD.[100]

Multimodal approaches emphasized the additional diagnostic value of combined MR imaging[101] or MR imaging/PET techniques including

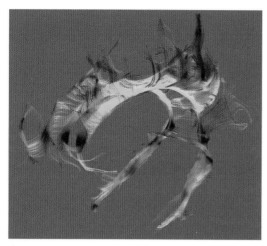

Fig. 12. Reconstruction of the entire cingulum bundles, including the parahippocampal cingulum, in a cognitively healthy elderly proband (70 years) using deterministic fibertractography. (*Courtesy of* Andreas Fellgiebel.)

DT imaging.[102] In addition, the specific contribution of DT imaging indices has been clarified: structural integrity measures such as fractional anisotropy, mean diffusivity, radial diffusivity, or axial diffusivity are not merely due to brain atrophy and are largely not easily exchangeable by other structural MR imaging measures.[103]

To date, contrary to diffusivity measurements in acute stroke, DT imaging has not entered the clinical routine. One reason for this is the lack of larger prospective multicenter studies to validate the diagnostic utility and the robustness of DT imaging in more naturalistic clinical settings. Second, automated imaging analyses have not been established as yet. However, the first European DTI Study in Dementia Group multicenter studies based on retrospective collection of DT imaging data from more than 330 subjects demonstrated acceptable multicenter and multiscanner effects of DT imaging indices as well as promising automated analyses.[104,105]

Frontal lobe myelination and connectivity, confirmed by neuropathologic, neuroradiologic, and functional studies, have been shown to play a key role in human brain development and degeneration.[98] In normal aging, a characteristic pattern of phenotypic motor and cognitive changes can be commonly observed, mainly resulting from reduced processing speed and decreased executive functioning.[106] More specifically, decreases in gait speed, psychomotor speed, reaction times, working memory, abstract reasoning, problem solving, and memory retrieval during the aging process provide evidence that frontal brain functions show the greatest vulnerability to decline in

normal aging. This regional cerebral aging pattern characterized by an anterior to posterior gradient of greater to lesser degeneration, could also be confirmed by several studies of structural connectivity using DT imaging.[107,108]

Age-related changes in white matter integrity as measured by DT imaging can be regarded as a surrogate of "cerebral disconnection," and could be associated with cognitive decline in normal aging. Decreases of structural white matter integrity within the superior parietal lobule pathway, the medial temporofrontal pathway, the uncinate fasciculus, the frontoparietal fasciculus, and the cingulum could be associated with decreased working memory function.[109]

It is suggested that structural integrity of the inferior longitudinal fasciculus may be associated with visuomotor function, the inferior occipitofrontal fasciculus is associated with visuospatial construction, and posterior corpus callosum fibers are associated with memory and executive function in normal aging.[110]

Initial studies suggest that DT imaging–derived measures of structural integrity or structural connectivity could yield surrogates of brain resilience or vulnerability in normal aging.

One study found an increased age-related decline in global and regional local interconnectivity in apolipoprotein E4 (ApoE4) carriers compared with noncarriers, indicating decreased structural network properties in subjects at risk of late-onset AD.[111] Moreover, a region-specific and function-specific influence of the ApoE genotype on the association between white matter integrity and cognitive function has been reported.[112] One study showed that higher education is associated with greater white matter integrity in medial temporal lobe areas and association fiber tracts.[113]

Using region-of-interest–based DT imaging analyses in AD or MCI, several studies demonstrated structural disturbances in brain, predominately in regions that are known to be preferentially affected or affected early in AD (hippocampal, temporal, posterior cingulate bundles, parietal).[114–124] Voxel-based analyses of DT imaging data consistently showed comparable results,[125,126] especially in that the white matter tracts within corpus callosum, the cingulum, and fornix, as well as the frontal and temporal white matter, seem to be affected early in AD. A meta-analysis of 41 DT imaging studies in individuals with AD and MCI (including a total of 2026 subjects) found significant decreases in fractional anisotrophy in AD subjects in comparison with controls, with good effect sizes in all analyzed regions (especially posterior cingulate bundles, splenium, temporal white matter, parahippocampal, uncinate fascicle, and superior longitudinal fascicle) except the parietal and occipital white matter.[127]

A combination of volume and diffusivity measurements might improve the diagnostic accuracy. The authors demonstrated enhanced prediction of episodic memory impairment when combining hippocampal volume and mean diffusivity measures in amnestic MCI subjects and healthy controls.[101]

The occurrence of global and regional volume reduction in the hippocampus has been a consistent finding of structural MR studies of AD patients, as well as in subjects with MCI. Studies investigating microstructural alterations of the hippocampus demonstrated a significant association of left anterior hippocampal diffusivity and verbal memory in early AD. Moreover, using a bimodal approach including DT imaging and FDG PET, a significant correlation between left anterior hippocampal mean diffusivity and relative FDG uptake was observed in patients with early AD.[102]

In a longitudinal observation study it was explored whether microstructural indices of hippocampal integrity can predict transition to dementia in subjects with MCI. Thirteen MCI patients were followed up by clinical assessment over a mean period of 1.5 years.[128] Patients who converted to dementia during the observation period had significantly elevated left hippocampal mean diffusivity at baseline compared with those MCI patients who remained clinically stable. This finding was independently obtained by another working group that also reported increased baseline hippocampal diffusivity as a predictor of conversion to dementia in MCI patients.[129]

DT imaging can already be regarded as a powerful new MR technique to sensitively quantify alterations of white matter integrity. The utility and feasibility of DT imaging for early AD diagnosis and for the monitoring (or treatment) of the disease needs further evaluation, especially in comparisons with other MR-measures and in the context of larger multicenter approaches.

Fibertractography, which allows one to reconstruct and quantify fiber connections, could qualify as a feasible new postprocessing tool for DT imaging data for automated analyses of functionally structural networks in normal aging in comparison with MCI and AD.[105,130] One further promising development is the combination of DT imaging with other imaging modalities, especially different PET modalities such as FDG PET[131,132] or amyloid PET, and fMR imaging.[132,133] The combination of these methods may help to improve our understanding of the interplay of AD-specific pathology, synaptic (dys-)function, and underlying network integrity, and thus detect the necessary conditions of upcoming clinical AD. There is early evidence that DT imaging might contribute to quantification of individual cognitive reserve,[113] suggesting that the multimodal approach might improve our knowledge on individual resilience and vulnerability to AD pathology on the imaging level.

ARTERIAL SPIN LABELING

Imaging of cerebral perfusion with ASL is a potentially very attractive diagnostic tool, owing to its noninvasiveness and rapid acquisition time. Technical challenges, such as small changes in signals of interest, are continuously addressed, and the reliability of the method is improving. In parallel, its application in AD and MCI has recently increased.

The pattern of hypoperfusion observed with ASL in AD is very similar to patterns of hypometabolism derived from FDG PET in AD patients.[134,135] Thus, areas of hypoperfusion in AD include the precuneus and parietal region as well as frontal regions.[136,137] Moreover, similar sensitivity and specificity for the discrimination between patients and controls have been suggested in pilot studies but require confirmation in larger studies, optimally including histopathologic postmortem assessment of the true extent of pathologic involvement.[137,138]

The perfusion in the cingulate in AD patients has been shown to increase after 12 weeks of treatment with donepezil, and this change correlated with clinical response to treatment.[139]

Regarding the medial temporal lobe, there are reports on reduced blood flow,[136] but also on increased perfusion after correction for atrophy.[140] This finding suggests that standard algorithms for handling atrophy are required to achieve reproducible results, which is a requirement for diagnostic application in the future.

In patients with MCI topographic patterns of hypoperfusion similar to, though less pronounced than those in AD patients have been observed.[134,136,141] Regarding the medial temporal lobe, there have also been reports on increased perfusion in MCI.[142] One longitudinal ASL study over 2.7 years reported prediction of conversion from MCI to dementia by hypoperfusion within the right inferior parietal and right middle frontal lobe.[143] Overall, the data on ASL in AD and MCI are rapidly growing, and clinical application in the diagnostic process of AD and MCI may be possible in the future.

PROTON MR SPECTROSCOPY

^{1}H MR spectroscopy provides information on the concentration of specific molecular groups (metabolites) in the brain tissue. The amino acid *N*-acetylaspartate (NAA) provides a highly reliable ^{1}H MR spectroscopy signal. NAA is a marker of neuronal density and of the functional state of neurons. Numerous studies have reported a reduction of the neuronal marker NAA in the brain tissue of AD patients.[144] The spatial distribution of NAA reduction in AD reflects the pattern of neuronal damage, with a pronounced reduction in the medial temporal lobe[145,146] and the posterior cingulate cortex/precuneus region.[147] Brain regions with only minor neuronal damage do not show NAA reduction.[148] Nevertheless, the NAA reduction and volume atrophy are not highly correlated, and the combination of NAA and volume measures in discriminating AD patients from healthy individuals is superior to either one alone.[146,149] The degree of NAA reduction is not stable over time in patients. In fact, several studies have shown increases of NAA under pharmacologic treatment.[150,151]

The second MR spectroscopic marker that is relevant for the distinction of AD patients from healthy individuals is myo-inositol, which is considered a glial marker. Myo-inositol is mostly increased in AD.[144] Some studies provide evidence that myo-inositol may be increased before NAA decreases in AD.[147]

Several studies have reported reduced NAA and increased myo-inositol as early as the MCI stage in cross-sectional investigations,[144] and have identified both as a predictor for conversion to AD, independent of volumetric measures (eg, Ref.[152]). In small studies, it has been shown that NAA is already reduced in mutation carriers of causal AD genes even at the asymptomatic stage.[153] Myo-inositol has also been found to increase in cognitively healthy individuals with positive amyloid labeling in PET.[154]

Today ^{1}H MR spectroscopy is standardized for clinical applications, but is still is not widely used in clinical practice. However, it can provide important information on biochemical aspects of the brain tissue, which is not provided by any other imaging technique, and may be particularly useful in early detection of disease.

FUNCTIONAL MR IMAGING ACTIVATION STUDIES

Task-related fMR imaging is increasingly used to study neuronal network dysfunction associated with AD. The majority of fMR imaging studies have used an episodic memory task to investigate the medial temporal lobe memory system. The studies consistently report reduced activation in the hippocampus and parahippocampal regions during encoding.[155] In addition, there is the common observation of reduced activation in frontal brain, the precuneus, and the cingulate gyrus. By contrast, increased activation of the prefrontal brain has been observed, and usually has been interpreted as increased compensatory neuronal activity.[156]

In those with MCI and healthy subjects at risk, the data are more varied. There is evidence that particularly the medial temporal lobe system is hyperactive during memory tasks in cognitively normal performing subjects who are at increased genetic risk (eg, ApoE4 carriers), whereas at the MCI stage, activation decreases and memory functions decline (eg, Refs.[157,158]). It has been suggested that increased activation of the medial temporal lobe system may be a predictor of more rapid decline.[159] A recent study showed that individuals with subjective memory impairment, but still normal performance, already show reduced hippocampal and increased prefrontal activation.[160] A further finding is the reduced ability to downregulate or deactivate nonrequired brain regions, which refers for example to activity in the default-mode network during encoding in AD and MCI patients.[155,161] Another previous study was able to demonstrate an inability to deactivate the auditory cortex during a visually demanding navigation task.[162]

Wermke and colleagues[163] provide a comprehensive review of activation and deactivation mechanisms in AD. In comparison with other MR modalities, cognitive fMR imaging is more prone to subject-related variations, which are caused by technical issues such as sensitivity to head-movement artifacts, and by patient-related issues such as comprehension of the respective tasks and vigilance, among others. These characteristics of cognitive fMR imaging limit its application as an individual diagnostic procedure. The strength of cognitive fMR imaging is the understanding of cognitive mechanisms within the course of the disease and, potentially, the assessment of functional effects of different treatments (eg, Ref.[164]).

RESTING-STATE FUNCTIONAL CONNECTIVITY

The continued development of novel sophisticated neuroimaging procedures allows assessment of functional brain networks in humans by means of resting-state fMR imaging. The most frequently investigated system is the so-called default-mode network. This network has been demonstrated to be active during internally focused cognitive processes, but deactivated during externally focused cognitive tasks. With regard to AD, the default-mode network is of interest with regard to several aspects. First, disconnection of default network regions has been demonstrated in very early stages of AD and even in MCI.[165] Second, a striking anatomic overlap has been shown between default network regions and the topographic distribution of different AD abnormalities, such as amyloid deposition, hypometabolism, and brain atrophy.[166] These findings have stimulated the discussion of a network-based expansion of neurodegenerative pathologic conditions.[167] A great advantage of resting-state fMR imaging over fMR imaging activation studies is the absence of any need for interaction of the patient, thus allowing better standardization and reproducibility. Together with the proof of very early abnormalities of network function in AD, these findings suggest that resting-state fMR imaging may potentially qualify as a diagnostic tool in the future.

MULTIMODAL APPROACHES

It can be summarized that today, several suitable neuroimaging procedures are available that capture different aspects of neurodegeneration. The various existing MR imaging procedures as well as modern PET methods such as amyloid imaging provide complementary information about pathophysiologic changes in the brain associated with neurodegeneration. In consequence, depending on the clinical question and the availability of the corresponding methods, a combination of several diagnostic tools may result in optimal diagnostic results. Indeed, several studies suggest superior performance of a combination of different imaging modalities.[168–170]

The discussion about the use of multimodal imaging approaches to improve diagnostic performance may gain even more momentum in the future with the introduction of the recently established hybrid PET/MR instrumentation in a single scanner. This hybrid imaging technology will allow acquisition of structural, functional, and molecular information in one session, and thus may significantly influence future diagnostic protocols.[171]

SUMMARY

Adequate diagnostic workup should be performed in every demented patient with clinical signs of dementia. Following thorough clinical examination and a survey of the patient's history, structural neuroimaging can be regarded as a mandatory subsequent step. The first important aim of brain imaging consists in the exclusion of non-neurodegenerative intracerebral conditions that may be potentially treatable even if they occur not exclusively but in addition to a neurodegenerative process (eg, vascular abnormalities). Routine MR imaging procedures discussed in this review offer optimal tools to catch a broad variety of non-neurodegenerative abnormalities potentially leading to cognitive impairment, and are thus important in preventing misdiagnosis. Neuroimaging, therefore, should be part of the diagnostic cascade, particularly in cases with atypical characteristics (eg, sudden onset or rapid progression of cognitive decline).[16]

After exclusion of non-neurodegenerative abnormality, the next information to be gleaned from imaging will consist of confirmation of a specific neurodegenerative disorder (eg, AD) or differential diagnosis from other forms. MR imaging may show inferior performance in this context in comparison with, for example, FDG PET. However, characteristic patterns of atrophy have been demonstrated in different forms of dementia and may certainly support the clinical diagnosis, particularly when PET methods are not available. Regarding early diagnosis of neurodegenerative disorders in mild or even asymptomatic stages, structural MR imaging is not regarded as the method of choice, based on the assumption that neuronal loss represents a somewhat late phenomenon of neurodegeneration. In this context, FDG PET has been demonstrated to be of higher value in the stage of MCI, and amyloid imaging may even allow detection of subjects with ongoing amyloid abnormality ahead of cognitive symptoms. However, with regard to longitudinal assessment, it has been shown that brain-volume loss over time may reliably detect subjects on their way to AD in the very early stages. Furthermore, longitudinal imaging may represent a highly valuable tool for therapy trials attempting to target neuronal loss as an end point of treatment success.

In addition to structural imaging, an impressive number of new MR imaging procedures are under evaluation, which may find their way into clinical application in the future. Such methods include the assessment of altered white matter integrity by means of DT imaging, the identification of regional hypoperfusion with ASL, and the monitoring of biochemical changes using ^{1}H MR spectroscopy. Furthermore, resting-state fMR imaging offers the fascinating opportunity to capture changes in function or dysfunction of neuronal networks. These tools may help to improve our understanding of disease pathophysiology and may become sensitive and specific biomarkers for early diagnosis and disease monitoring in the future.

Most imaging tools discussed in this review provide complementary information on different aspects on disease pathology. Thus, the selection of the appropriate imaging tool is highly dependent on the actual diagnostic question. Furthermore, the combination of several of the imaging biomarkers mentioned may lead to an optimal diagnostic result. The introduction of hybrid imaging technology such as PET/MR may pave the way for such a multimodal imaging approach.

REFERENCES

1. Blennow K, de Leon MJ, Zetterberg H. Alzheimer's disease. Lancet 2006;368(9533):387–403.

2. Bickel H. Dementia syndrome and Alzheimer disease: an assessment of morbidity and annual incidence in Germany. Gesundheitswesen 2000;62(4): 211–8 [in German].

3. Hebert LE, Scherr PA, Bienias JL, et al. Alzheimer disease in the US population: prevalence estimates using the 2000 census. Arch Neurol 2003;60(8): 1119–22.

4. Plassman BL, Langa KM, Fisher GG, et al. Prevalence of dementia in the United States: the aging, demographics, and memory study. Neuroepidemiology 2007;29(1–2):125–32.

5. Braak E, Griffing K, Arai K, et al. Neuropathology of Alzheimer's disease: what is new since A. Alzheimer? Eur Arch Psychiatry Clin Neurosci 1999; 249(Suppl 3):14–22.

6. Davies L, Wolska B, Hilbich C, et al. A4 amyloid protein deposition and the diagnosis of Alzheimer's disease: prevalence in aged brains determined by immunocytochemistry compared with conventional neuropathologic techniques. Neurology 1988; 38(11):1688–93.

7. Petersen RC. Mild cognitive impairment as a diagnostic entity. J Intern Med 2004;256(3):183–94.

8. Forstl H, Kurz A. Clinical features of Alzheimer's disease. Eur Arch Psychiatry Clin Neurosci 1999; 249(6):288–90.

9. McKhann G, Drachman D, Folstein M, et al. Clinical diagnosis of Alzheimer's disease: report of the NINCDS-ADRDA Work Group under the auspices of Department of Health and Human Services Task Force on Alzheimer's Disease. Neurology 1984;34(7):939–44.

10. Hull M, Berger M, Heneka M. Disease-modifying therapies in Alzheimer's disease: how far have we come? Drugs 2006;66(16):2075–93.

11. Sperling RA, Aisen PS, Beckett LA, et al. Toward defining the preclinical stages of Alzheimer's disease: recommendations from the National Institute on Aging-Alzheimer's Association workgroups on diagnostic guidelines for Alzheimer's disease. Alzheimers Dement 2011;7(3):280–92.

12. Albert MS, DeKosky ST, Dickson D, et al. The diagnosis of mild cognitive impairment due to Alzheimer's disease: recommendations from the National Institute on Aging-Alzheimer's Association workgroups on diagnostic guidelines for Alzheimer's disease. Alzheimers Dement 2011;7(3): 270–9.

13. McKhann GM, Knopman DS, Chertkow H, et al. The diagnosis of dementia due to Alzheimer's disease: recommendations from the National Institute on Aging-Alzheimer's Association workgroups on diagnostic guidelines for Alzheimer's disease. Alzheimers Dement 2011;7(3):263–9.

14. Dubois B, Feldman HH, Jacova C, et al. Research criteria for the diagnosis of Alzheimer's disease: revising the NINCDS-ADRDA criteria. Lancet Neurol 2007;6(8):734–46.

15. Yuan Y, Gu ZX, Wei WS. Fluorodeoxyglucose-positron-emission tomography, single-photon emission tomography, and structural MR imaging for prediction of rapid conversion to Alzheimer disease in patients with mild cognitive impairment: a meta-analysis. AJNR Am J Neuroradiol 2009;30(2): 404–10.

16. Geschwind MD, Shu H, Haman A, et al. Rapidly progressive dementia. Ann Neurol 2008;64(1):97–108.

17. Lee SH, Kim SM, Kim N, et al. Cortico-subcortical distribution of microbleeds is different between hypertension and cerebral amyloid angiopathy. J Neurol Sci 2007;258(1–2):111–4.

18. Cavalieri M, Schmidt H, Schmidt R. Structural MRI in normal aging and Alzheimer's disease: white and black spots. Neurodegener Dis 2012;10(1–4): 253–6.

19. Shiga Y, Miyazawa K, Sato S, et al. Diffusion-weighted MRI abnormalities as an early diagnostic marker for Creutzfeldt-Jakob disease. Neurology 2004;63(3):443–9.

20. Baringer JR. Herpes simplex infections of the nervous system. Neurol Clin 2008;26(3):657–74, viii.

21. Hatipoglu HG, Sakman B, Yuksel E. Magnetic resonance and diffusion-weighted imaging findings of herpes simplex encephalitis. Herpes 2008;15(1): 13–7.

22. Filippi M, Rocca MA. Conventional MRI in multiple sclerosis. J Neuroimaging 2007;17(Suppl 1):3S–9S.

23. Traboulsee AL, Li DK. The role of MRI in the diagnosis of multiple sclerosis. Adv Neurol 2006;98: 125–46.

24. Polman CH, Reingold SC, Edan G, et al. Diagnostic criteria for multiple sclerosis: 2005 revisions to the "McDonald Criteria". Ann Neurol 2005;58(6):840–6.

25. van der Lijn F, den Heijer T, Breteler MM, et al. Hippocampus segmentation in MR images using atlas registration, voxel classification, and graph cuts. Neuroimage 2008;43(4):708–20.

26. Ashburner J, Friston KJ. Voxel-based morphometry—the methods. Neuroimage 2000;11(6 Pt 1): 805–21.

27. Querbes O, Aubry F, Pariente J, et al. Early diagnosis of Alzheimer's disease using cortical thickness: impact of cognitive reserve. Brain 2009; 132(Pt 8):2036–47.

28. Lerch JP, Pruessner J, Zijdenbos AP, et al. Automated cortical thickness measurements from MRI can accurately separate Alzheimer's patients from normal elderly controls. Neurobiol Aging 2008; 29(1):23–30.

29. Lerch JP, Pruessner JC, Zijdenbos A, et al. Focal decline of cortical thickness in Alzheimer's disease identified by computational neuroanatomy. Cereb Cortex 2005;15(7):995–1001.

30. Scheltens P, Leys D, Barkhof F, et al. Atrophy of medial temporal lobes on MRI in "probable" Alzheimer's disease and normal ageing: diagnostic value and neuropsychological correlates. J Neurol Neurosurg Psychiatry 1992;55(10):967–72.

31. Pasquier F, Leys D, Weerts JG, et al. Inter- and intraobserver reproducibility of cerebral atrophy assessment on MRI scans with hemispheric infarcts. Eur Neurol 1996;36(5):268–72.

32. Wattjes MP. Structural MRI. Int Psychogeriatr 2011; 23(Suppl 2):S13–24.

33. Drzezga A. Diagnosis of Alzheimer's disease with [18F]PET in mild and asymptomatic stages. Behav Neurol 2009;21(1):101–15.

34. Drzezga A, Grimmer T, Riemenschneider M, et al. Prediction of individual clinical outcome in MCI by means of genetic assessment and (18)F-FDG PET. J Nucl Med 2005;46(10):1625–32.

35. Silverman DH, Small GW, Chang CY, et al. Positron emission tomography in evaluation of dementia: regional brain metabolism and long-term outcome. JAMA 2001;286(17):2120–7.

36. Minoshima S, Giordani B, Berent S, et al. Metabolic reduction in the posterior cingulate cortex in very early Alzheimer's disease. Ann Neurol 1997;42(1): 85–94.

37. Drzezga A. Amyloid-plaque imaging in early and differential diagnosis of dementia. Ann Nucl Med 2010;24:55–66.

38. Li TQ, Wahlund LO. The search for neuroimaging biomarkers of Alzheimer's disease with advanced MRI techniques. Acta Radiol 2011;52(2):211–22.

39. Wolk DA, Detre JA. Arterial spin labeling MRI: an emerging biomarker for Alzheimer's disease and other neurodegenerative conditions. Curr Opin Neurol 2012;25(4):421–8.

40. Tartaglia MC, Rosen HJ, Miller BL. Neuroimaging in dementia. Neurotherapeutics 2011;8(1):82–92.

41. Minati L, Grisoli M, Bruzzone MG. MR spectroscopy, functional MRI, and diffusion-tensor imaging in the aging brain: a conceptual review. J Geriatr Psychiatry Neurol 2007;20(1):3–21.

42. Brand A, Richter-Landsberg C, Leibfritz D. Multinuclear NMR studies on the energy metabolism of glial and neuronal cells. Dev Neurosci 1993; 15(3–5):289–98.

43. Buckner RL, Andrews-Hanna JR, Schacter DL. The brain's default network: anatomy, function, and relevance to disease. Ann N Y Acad Sci 2008; 1124:1–38.

44. Biswal B, Yetkin FZ, Haughton VM, et al. Functional connectivity in the motor cortex of resting human brain using echo-planar MRI. Magn Reson Med 1995;34(4):537–41.

45. Greicius MD, Krasnow B, Reiss AL, et al. Functional connectivity in the resting brain: a network analysis of the default mode hypothesis. Proc Natl Acad Sci U S A 2003;100(1):253–8.

46. Greicius MD, Srivastava G, Reiss AL, et al. Default-mode network activity distinguishes Alzheimer's disease from healthy aging: evidence from functional MRI. Proc Natl Acad Sci U S A 2004; 101(13):4637–42.

47. Rombouts SA, Barkhof F, Goekoop R, et al. Altered resting state networks in mild cognitive impairment and mild Alzheimer's disease: an fMRI study. Hum Brain Mapp 2005;26(4):231–9.

48. Garrity AG, Pearlson GD, McKiernan K, et al. Aberrant "default mode" functional connectivity in schizophrenia. Am J Psychiatry 2007;164(3): 450–7.

49. Harrison BJ, Yucel M, Pujol J, et al. Task-induced deactivation of midline cortical regions in schizophrenia assessed with fMRI. Schizophr Res 2007; 91(1–3):82–6.

50. Kennedy DP, Redcay E, Courchesne E. Failing to deactivate: resting functional abnormalities in autism. Proc Natl Acad Sci U S A 2006;103(21): 8275–80.

51. Kapeller P, Schmidt R, Fazekas F. Qualitative MRI: evidence of usual aging in the brain. Top Magn Reson Imaging 2004;15(6):343–7.

52. Fazekas F, Chawluk JB, Alavi A, et al. MR signal abnormalities at 1.5 T in Alzheimer's dementia and normal aging. AJR Am J Roentgenol 1987; 149(2):351–6.

53. Heier LA, Bauer CJ, Schwartz L, et al. Large Virchow-Robin spaces: MR-clinical correlation. AJNR Am J Neuroradiol 1989;10(5):929–36.

54. Jack CR Jr, Lowe VJ, Weigand SD, et al. Serial PIB and MRI in normal, mild cognitive impairment and Alzheimer's disease: implications for sequence of pathological events in Alzheimer's disease. Brain 2009;132(Pt 5):1355–65.

55. Raz N, Rodrigue KM, Head D, et al. Differential aging of the medial temporal lobe: a study of a five-year change. Neurology 2004;62(3):433–8.

56. Tabert MH, Manly JJ, Liu X, et al. Neuropsychological prediction of conversion to Alzheimer disease in patients with mild cognitive impairment. Arch Gen Psychiatry 2006;63(8):916–24.

57. Petersen RC, Smith GE, Waring SC, et al. Mild cognitive impairment: clinical characterization and outcome. Arch Neurol 1999;56(3):303–8.

58. Jack CR Jr, Petersen RC, Xu YC, et al. Prediction of AD with MRI-based hippocampal volume in mild cognitive impairment. Neurology 1999;52(7):1397–403.

59. Wang PN, Lirng JF, Lin KN, et al. Prediction of Alzheimer's disease in mild cognitive impairment: a prospective study in Taiwan. Neurobiol Aging 2006;27(12):1797–806.

60. Pennanen C, Testa C, Laakso MP, et al. A voxel based morphometry study on mild cognitive impairment. J Neurol Neurosurg Psychiatry 2005; 76(1):11–4.

61. Du AT, Schuff N, Amend D, et al. Magnetic resonance imaging of the entorhinal cortex and hippocampus in mild cognitive impairment and Alzheimer's disease. J Neurol Neurosurg Psychiatry 2001;71(4):441–7.

62. Hampel H, Burger K, Teipel SJ, et al. Core candidate neurochemical and imaging biomarkers of Alzheimer's disease. Alzheimers Dement 2008; 4(1):38–48.

63. Chetelat G, Desgranges B, De La Sayette V, et al. Mapping gray matter loss with voxel-based morphometry in mild cognitive impairment. Neuroreport 2002;13(15):1939–43.

64. Singh V, Chertkow H, Lerch JP, et al. Spatial patterns of cortical thinning in mild cognitive impairment and Alzheimer's disease. Brain 2006; 129(Pt 11):2885–93.

65. Jack CR Jr, Petersen RC, Xu YC, et al. Medial temporal atrophy on MRI in normal aging and very mild Alzheimer's disease. Neurology 1997;49(3): 786–94.

66. Fox NC, Warrington EK, Freeborough PA, et al. Presymptomatic hippocampal atrophy in Alzheimer's disease. A longitudinal MRI study. Brain 1996; 119(Pt 6):2001–7.

67. Jack CR Jr, Shiung MM, Gunter JL, et al. Comparison of different MRI brain atrophy rate measures with clinical disease progression in AD. Neurology 2004;62(4):591–600.

68. Gosche KM, Mortimer JA, Smith CD, et al. Hippocampal volume as an index of Alzheimer neuropathology: findings from the Nun Study. Neurology 2002;58(10):1476–82.

69. Du AT, Schuff N, Kramer JH, et al. Higher atrophy rate of entorhinal cortex than hippocampus in AD. Neurology 2004;62(3):422–7.

70. Wahlund LO, Julin P, Johansson SE, et al. Visual rating and volumetry of the medial temporal lobe on magnetic resonance imaging in dementia: a comparative study. J Neurol Neurosurg Psychiatry 2000;69(5):630–5.

71. Seelaar H, Rohrer JD, Pijnenburg YA, et al. Clinical, genetic and pathological heterogeneity of frontotemporal dementia: a review. J Neurol Neurosurg Psychiatry 2011;82(5):476–86.

72. Rohrer JD, Rosen HJ. Neuroimaging in frontotemporal dementia. Int Rev Psychiatry 2013;25(2):221–9.

73. Gorno-Tempini ML, Dronkers NF, Rankin KP, et al. Cognition and anatomy in three variants of primary progressive aphasia. Ann Neurol 2004; 55(3):335–46.

74. Burton EJ, Karas G, Paling SM, et al. Patterns of cerebral atrophy in dementia with Lewy bodies using voxel-based morphometry. Neuroimage 2002; 17(2):618–30.

75. Jack CR Jr, Petersen RC, Xu Y, et al. Rate of medial temporal lobe atrophy in typical aging and Alzheimer's disease. Neurology 1998;51(4):993–9.

76. Laakso MP, Lehtovirta M, Partanen K, et al. Hippocampus in Alzheimer's disease: a 3-year follow-up MRI study. Biol Psychiatry 2000;47(6):557–61.

77. Frisoni GB, Fox NC, Jack CR Jr, et al. The clinical use of structural MRI in Alzheimer disease. Nat Rev Neurol 2010;6(2):67–77.

78. Baron JC, Chetelat G, Desgranges B, et al. In vivo mapping of gray matter loss with voxel-based morphometry in mild Alzheimer's disease. Neuroimage 2001;14(2):298–309.

79. Busatto GF, Garrido GE, Almeida OP, et al. A voxel-based morphometry study of temporal lobe gray matter reductions in Alzheimer's disease. Neurobiol Aging 2003;24(2):221–31.

80. Bocti C, Rockel C, Roy P, et al. Topographical patterns of lobar atrophy in frontotemporal dementia and Alzheimer's disease. Dement Geriatr Cogn Disord 2006;21(5–6):364–72.

81. Rabinovici GD, Seeley WW, Kim EJ, et al. Distinct MRI atrophy patterns in autopsy-proven Alzheimer's disease and frontotemporal lobar degeneration. Am J Alzheimers Dis Other Demen 2007–2008;22(6):474–88.

82. Knopman DS, DeKosky ST, Cummings JL, et al. Practice parameter: diagnosis of dementia (an evidence-based review). Report of the Quality Standards Subcommittee of the American Academy of Neurology. Neurology 2001;56(9):1143–53.

83. Barber R, Scheltens P, Gholkar A, et al. White matter lesions on magnetic resonance imaging in dementia with Lewy bodies, Alzheimer's disease, vascular dementia, and normal aging. J Neurol Neurosurg Psychiatry 1999;67(1):66–72.

84. Scheltens P, Barkhof F, Valk J, et al. White matter lesions on magnetic resonance imaging in clinically diagnosed Alzheimer's disease. Evidence for heterogeneity. Brain 1992;115(Pt 3):735–48.

85. Burton EJ, McKeith IG, Burn DJ, et al. Progression of white matter hyperintensities in Alzheimer disease, dementia with Lewy bodies, and Parkinson disease dementia: a comparison with normal aging. Am J Geriatr Psychiatry 2006;14(10):842–9.

86. Holland CM, Smith EE, Csapo I, et al. Spatial distribution of white-matter hyperintensities in Alzheimer disease, cerebral amyloid angiopathy, and healthy aging. Stroke 2008;39(4):1127–33.

87. Pettersen JA, Sathiyamoorthy G, Gao FQ, et al. Microbleed topography, leukoaraiosis, and cognition in probable Alzheimer disease from the Sunnybrook dementia study. Arch Neurol 2008;65(6): 790–5.

88. Carmichael O, Schwarz C, Drucker D, et al. Longitudinal changes in white matter disease and cognition in the first year of the Alzheimer disease neuroimaging initiative. Arch Neurol 2010;67(11): 1370–8.

89. Cordonnier C, Al-Shahi Salman R, Wardlaw J. Spontaneous brain microbleeds: systematic review, subgroup analyses and standards for study design and reporting. Brain 2007;130(Pt 8):1988–2003.

90. van der Flier WM. Clinical aspects of microbleeds in Alzheimer's disease. J Neurol Sci 2012;322(1–2): 56–8.

91. Cordonnier C, van der Flier WM. Brain microbleeds and Alzheimer's disease: innocent observation or key player? Brain 2011;134(Pt 2):335–44.

92. Goos JD, Kester MI, Barkhof F, et al. Patients with Alzheimer disease with multiple microbleeds: relation with cerebrospinal fluid biomarkers and cognition. Stroke 2009;40(11):3455–60.

93. Sjobeck M, Haglund M, Englund E. White matter mapping in Alzheimer's disease: a neuropathological study. Neurobiol Aging 2006;27(5):673–80.

94. Sjobeck M, Haglund M, Englund E. Decreasing myelin density reflected increasing white matter pathology in Alzheimer's disease—a neuropathological study. Int J Geriatr Psychiatry 2005;20(10): 919–26.

95. Gouw AA, Seewann A, Vrenken H, et al. Heterogeneity of white matter hyperintensities in Alzheimer's disease: post-mortem quantitative MRI and neuropathology. Brain 2008;131(Pt 12):3286–98.

96. Bartzokis G. Age-related myelin breakdown: a developmental model of cognitive decline and Alzheimer's disease. Neurobiol Aging 2004;25(1):5–18 [author reply: 49–62].

97. Bartzokis G, Cummings JL, Sultzer D, et al. White matter structural integrity in healthy aging adults and patients with Alzheimer disease: a magnetic resonance imaging study. Arch Neurol 2003; 60(3):393–8.

98. Sherin J, Bartzokis G. Human brain myelination trajectories across the fife span: Implications for CNS function and dysfunction. In: Masoro EJ, Austad SN, editors. Handbook of the biology of aging. 7th edition. London: Elsevier; 2011. p. 333–46.

99. De Reuck J, Deramecourt V, Cordonnier C, et al. The impact of cerebral amyloid angiopathy on the occurrence of cerebrovascular lesions in demented patients with Alzheimer features: a neuropathological study. Eur J Neurol 2011;18(6): 913–8.

100. Avants BB, Cook PA, Ungar L, et al. Dementia induces correlated reductions in white matter integrity and cortical thickness: a multivariate neuroimaging study with sparse canonical correlation analysis. Neuroimage 2010;50(3):1004–16.

101. Müller MJ, Greverus D, Dellani PR, et al. Functional implications of hippocampal volume and diffusivity in mild cognitive impairment. Neuroimage 2005; 28(4):1033–42.

102. Fellgiebel A, Yakushev I. Diffusion tensor imaging of the hippocampus in MCI and early Alzheimer's disease. J Alzheimers Dis 2011; 26(Suppl 3):257–62.

103. Hugenschmidt CE, Peiffer AM, Kraft RA, et al. Relating imaging indices of white matter integrity and volume in healthy older adults. Cereb Cortex 2008;18(2):433–42.

104. Teipel SJ, Reuter S, Stieltjes B, et al. Multicenter stability of diffusion tensor imaging measures: a European clinical and physical phantom study. Psychiatry Res 2011;194(3):363–71.

105. Fischer FU, Scheurich A, Wegrzyn M, et al. Automated tractography of the cingulate bundle in Alzheimer's disease: a multicenter DTI study. J Magn Reson Imaging 2012;36(1):84–91.

106. Pugh KG, Lipsitz LA. The microvascular frontal-subcortical syndrome of aging. Neurobiol Aging 2002;23(3):421–31.

107. Michielse S, Coupland N, Camicioli R, et al. Selective effects of aging on brain white matter microstructure: a diffusion tensor imaging tractography study. Neuroimage 2010;52(4):1190–201.

108. Sullivan EV, Rohlfing T, Pfefferbaum A. Longitudinal study of callosal microstructure in the normal adult aging brain using quantitative DTI fiber tracking. Dev Neuropsychol 2010;35(3):233–56.

109. Charlton RA, Barrick TR, Lawes IN, et al. White matter pathways associated with working memory in normal aging. Cortex 2010;46(4):474–89.

110. Voineskos AN, Rajji TK, Lobaugh NJ, et al. Age-related decline in white matter tract integrity and cognitive performance: a DTI tractography and structural equation modeling study. Neurobiol Aging 2012;33(1):21–34.

111. Brown JA, Terashima KH, Burggren AC, et al. Brain network local interconnectivity loss in aging APOE-4 allele carriers. Proc Natl Acad Sci U S A 2011;108(51):20760–5.

112. Bartzokis G, Lu PH, Geschwind DH, et al. Apolipoprotein E affects both myelin breakdown and cognition: implications for age-related trajectories of decline into dementia. Biol Psychiatry 2007; 62(12):1380–7.

113. Teipel SJ, Meindl T, Wagner M, et al. White matter microstructure in relation to education in aging and Alzheimer's disease. J Alzheimers Dis 2009; 17(3):571–83.

114. Hanyu H, Sakurai H, Iwamoto T, et al. Diffusion-weighted MR imaging of the hippocampus and temporal white matter in Alzheimer's disease. J Neurol Sci 1998;156(2):195–200.

115. Bozzali M, Franceschi M, Falini A, et al. Quantification of tissue damage in AD using diffusion tensor and magnetization transfer MRI. Neurology 2001; 57(6):1135–7.

116. Zhang Y, Schuff N, Jahng GH, et al. Diffusion tensor imaging of cingulum fibers in mild cognitive impairment and Alzheimer disease. Neurology 2007;68(1):13–9.

117. Bozzali M, Falini A, Franceschi M, et al. White matter damage in Alzheimer's disease assessed in vivo using diffusion tensor magnetic resonance imaging. J Neurol Neurosurg Psychiatry 2002; 72(6):742–6.

118. Yoshiura T, Mihara F, Ogomori K, et al. Diffusion tensor in posterior cingulate gyrus: correlation with cognitive decline in Alzheimer's disease. Neuroreport 2002;13(17):2299–302.

119. Takahashi S, Yonezawa H, Takahashi J, et al. Selective reduction of diffusion anisotropy in white matter of Alzheimer disease brains measured by 3.0 Tesla magnetic resonance imaging. Neurosci Lett 2002; 332(1):45–8.

120. Rose SE, Chen F, Chalk JB, et al. Loss of connectivity in Alzheimer's disease: an evaluation of white matter tract integrity with colour coded MR diffusion tensor imaging. J Neurol Neurosurg Psychiatry 2000;69(4):528–30.

121. Fellgiebel A, Wille P, Muller MJ, et al. Ultrastructural hippocampal and white matter alterations in mild cognitive impairment: a diffusion tensor imaging study. Dement Geriatr Cogn Disord 2004;18(1): 101–8.

122. Fellgiebel A, Muller MJ, Wille P, et al. Color-coded diffusion-tensor-imaging of posterior cingulate fiber tracts in mild cognitive impairment. Neurobiol Aging 2005;26(8):1193–8.

123. Kantarci K, Jack CR Jr, Xu YC, et al. Mild cognitive impairment and Alzheimer disease: regional diffusivity of water. Radiology 2001;219(1):101–7.

124. Kalus P, Slotboom J, Gallinat J, et al. Examining the gateway to the limbic system with diffusion tensor imaging: the perforant pathway in dementia. Neuroimage 2006;30(3):713–20.

125. Teipel SJ, Stahl R, Dietrich O, et al. Multivariate network analysis of fiber tract integrity in Alzheimer's disease. Neuroimage 2007;34(3):985–95.

126. Xie S, Xiao JX, Gong GL, et al. Voxel-based detection of white matter abnormalities in mild Alzheimer disease. Neurology 2006;66(12):1845–9.

127. Sexton CE, Kalu UG, Filippini N, et al. A meta-analysis of diffusion tensor imaging in mild cognitive impairment and Alzheimer's disease. Neurobiol Aging 2011;32(12):2322.e5–18.

128. Fellgiebel A, Dellani PR, Greverus D, et al. Predicting conversion to dementia in mild cognitive impairment by volumetric and diffusivity measurements of the hippocampus. Psychiatry Res 2006;146(3): 283–7.

129. Kantarci K, Petersen RC, Boeve BF, et al. DWI predicts future progression to Alzheimer disease in amnestic mild cognitive impairment. Neurology 2005;64(5):902–4.

130. Lo CY, Wang PN, Chou KH, et al. Diffusion tensor tractography reveals abnormal topological organization in structural cortical networks in Alzheimer's disease. J Neurosci 2010;30(50): 16876–85.

131. Yakushev I, Gerhard A, Muller MJ, et al. Relationships between hippocampal microstructure, metabolism, and function in early Alzheimer's disease. Brain Struct Funct 2011;216(3):219–26.

132. Chetelat G, Landeau B, Salmon E, et al. Relationships between brain metabolism decrease in normal aging and changes in structural and functional connectivity. Neuroimage 2013;76:167–77.

133. Teipel SJ, Bokde AL, Meindl T, et al. White matter microstructure underlying default mode network connectivity in the human brain. Neuroimage 2010;49(3):2021–32.

134. Johnson NA, Jahng GH, Weiner MW, et al. Pattern of cerebral hypoperfusion in Alzheimer disease and mild cognitive impairment measured with arterial spin-labeling MR imaging: initial experience. Radiology 2005;234(3):851–9.

135. Asllani I, Habeck C, Scarmeas N, et al. Multivariate and univariate analysis of continuous arterial spin labeling perfusion MRI in Alzheimer's disease. J Cereb Blood Flow Metab 2008;28(4):725–36.

136. Alexopoulos P, Sorg C, Forschler A, et al. Perfusion abnormalities in mild cognitive impairment and mild dementia in Alzheimer's disease measured by pulsed arterial spin labeling MRI. Eur Arch Psychiatry Clin Neurosci 2012;262(1):69–77.

137. Musiek ES, Chen Y, Korczykowski M, et al. Direct comparison of fluorodeoxyglucose positron emission tomography and arterial spin labeling magnetic resonance imaging in Alzheimer's disease. Alzheimers Dement 2012;8(1):51–9.

138. Chen Y, Wolk DA, Reddin JS, et al. Voxel-level comparison of arterial spin-labeled perfusion MRI and FDG-PET in Alzheimer disease. Neurology 2011; 77(22):1977–85.

139. Li W, Antuono PG, Xie C, et al. Changes in regional cerebral blood flow and functional connectivity in the cholinergic pathway associated with cognitive performance in subjects with mild Alzheimer's

disease after 12-week donepezil treatment. Neuroimage 2012;60(2):1083–91.

140. Alsop DC, Casement M, de Bazelaire C, et al. Hippocampal hyperperfusion in Alzheimer's disease. Neuroimage 2008;42(4):1267–74.

141. Binnewijzend MA, Kuijer JP, Benedictus MR, et al. Cerebral blood flow measured with 3D pseudocontinuous arterial spin-labeling MR imaging in Alzheimer disease and mild cognitive impairment: a marker for disease severity. Radiology 2013; 267(1):221–30.

142. Dai W, Lopez OL, Carmichael OT, et al. Mild cognitive impairment and Alzheimer disease: patterns of altered cerebral blood flow at MR imaging. Radiology 2009;250(3):856–66.

143. Chao LL, Buckley ST, Kornak J, et al. ASL perfusion MRI predicts cognitive decline and conversion from MCI to dementia. Alzheimer Dis Assoc Disord 2010;24(1):19–27.

144. Kantarci K. [1]H magnetic resonance spectroscopy in dementia. Br J Radiol 2007;80(Spec No 2):S146–52.

145. Jessen F, Gur O, Block W, et al. A multicenter (1)H-MRS study of the medial temporal lobe in AD and MCI. Neurology 2009;72(20):1735–40.

146. Schuff N, Capizzano AA, Du AT, et al. Selective reduction of N-acetylaspartate in medial temporal and parietal lobes in AD. Neurology 2002;58(6): 928–35.

147. Kantarci K, Jack CR Jr, Xu YC, et al. Regional metabolic patterns in mild cognitive impairment and Alzheimer's disease: a ^{1}H MRS study. Neurology 2000;55(2):210–7.

148. Block W, Jessen F, Traber F, et al. Regional N-acetylaspartate reduction in the hippocampus detected with fast proton magnetic resonance spectroscopic imaging in patients with Alzheimer disease. Arch Neurol 2002;59(5):828–34.

149. Jessen F, Traeber F, Freymann N, et al. A comparative study of the different N-acetylaspartate measures of the medial temporal lobe in Alzheimer's disease. Dement Geriatr Cogn Disord 2005;20(2–3):178–83.

150. Krishnan KR, Charles HC, Doraiswamy PM, et al. Randomized, placebo-controlled trial of the effects of donepezil on neuronal markers and hippocampal volumes in Alzheimer's disease. Am J Psychiatry 2003;160(11):2003–11.

151. Jessen F, Traeber F, Freymann K, et al. Treatment monitoring and response prediction with proton MR spectroscopy in AD. Neurology 2006;67(3):528–30.

152. Metastasio A, Rinaldi P, Tarducci R, et al. Conversion of MCI to dementia: role of proton magnetic resonance spectroscopy. Neurobiol Aging 2006; 27(7):926–32.

153. Godbolt AK, Waldman AD, MacManus DG, et al. MRS shows abnormalities before symptoms in familial Alzheimer disease. Neurology 2006;66(5):718–22.

154. Kantarci K, Lowe V, Przybelski SA, et al. Magnetic resonance spectroscopy, beta-amyloid load, and cognition in a population-based sample of cognitively normal older adults. Neurology 2011;77(10): 951–8.

155. Sperling R. Potential of functional MRI as a biomarker in early Alzheimer's disease. Neurobiol Aging 2011;32(Suppl 1):S37–43.

156. Schwindt GC, Black SE. Functional imaging studies of episodic memory in Alzheimer's disease: a quantitative meta-analysis. Neuroimage 2009; 45(1):181–90.

157. Bookheimer SY, Strojwas MH, Cohen MS, et al. Patterns of brain activation in people at risk for Alzheimer's disease. N Engl J Med 2000;343(7): 450–6.

158. Johnson SC, Schmitz TW, Moritz CH, et al. Activation of brain regions vulnerable to Alzheimer's disease: the effect of mild cognitive impairment. Neurobiol Aging 2006;27(11):1604–12.

159. Sperling RA, Dickerson BC, Pihlajamaki M, et al. Functional alterations in memory networks in early Alzheimer's disease. Neuromolecular Med 2010; 12(1):27–43.

160. Erk S, Spottke A, Meisen A, et al. Evidence of neuronal compensation during episodic memory in subjective memory impairment. Arch Gen Psychiatry 2011;68(8):845–52.

161. Schwindt GC, Chaudhary S, Crane D, et al. Modulation of the default-mode network between rest and task in Alzheimer's disease. Cereb Cortex 2012;23(7):1685–94.

162. Drzezga A, Grimmer T, Peller M, et al. Impaired cross-modal inhibition in Alzheimer disease. PLoS Med 2005;2(10):e288.

163. Wermke M, Sorg C, Wohlschlager AM, et al. A new integrative model of cerebral activation, deactivation and default mode function in Alzheimer's disease. Eur J Nucl Med Mol Imaging 2008;35(Suppl 1):S12–24.

164. Bokde AL, Karmann M, Teipel SJ, et al. Decreased activation along the dorsal visual pathway after a 3-month treatment with galantamine in mild Alzheimer disease: a functional magnetic resonance imaging study. J Clin Psychopharmacol 2009; 29(2):147–56.

165. Sorg C, Riedl V, Muhlau M, et al. Selective changes of resting-state networks in individuals at risk for Alzheimer's disease. Proc Natl Acad Sci U S A 2007;104(47):18760–5.

166. Drzezga A, Becker JA, Van Dijk KR, et al. Neuronal dysfunction and disconnection of cortical hubs in non-demented subjects with elevated amyloid burden. Brain 2011;134(Pt 6):1635–46.

167. Seeley WW, Crawford RK, Zhou J, et al. Neurodegenerative diseases target large-scale human brain networks. Neuron 2009;62(1):42–52.

168. Jack CR Jr, Lowe VJ, Senjem ML, et al. [11]C PiB and structural MRI provide complementary information in imaging of Alzheimer's disease and amnestic mild cognitive impairment. Brain 2008;131(Pt 3):665–80.

169. Walhovd KB, Fjell AM, Amlien I, et al. Multimodal imaging in mild cognitive impairment: metabolism, morphometry and diffusion of the temporal-parietal memory network. Neuroimage 2008;45(1):215–23.

170. Kawachi T, Ishii K, Sakamoto S, et al. Comparison of the diagnostic performance of FDG-PET and VBM-MRI in very mild Alzheimer's disease. Eur J Nucl Med Mol Imaging 2006; 33(7):801–9.

171. Catana C, Drzezga A, Heiss WD, et al. PET/MRI for neurologic applications. J Nucl Med 2012;53(12): 1916–25.

Amyloid PET Imaging: MCI and AD

Vladimir Kepe, PhD

KEYWORDS

- Alzheimer disease • Mild cognitive impairment • Positron emission tomography
- "β-amyloid–specific" probes • Imaging biomarkers

KEY POINTS

- PET with "β-amyloid–specific" molecular imaging probes is a method developed in the past decade.
- Their use is proposed for the measurement of brain β-amyloid protein amyloidosis in the new guidelines for diagnosis of Alzheimer disease (AD) at different levels of disease progression.
- This article discusses limitations of this proposed use pointing to a number of unresolved issues and inconsistencies between PET scan results and correlation with other biomarkers, and with postmortem histopathological studies.
- These unresolved issues do not warrant the conclusion that PET imaging with "β-amyloid–specific" molecular imaging probes can be used as a biomarker in AD or in the various stages of disease progression.

INTRODUCTION

The Alzheimer disease (AD) research field has witnessed significant new developments in the past decade. Imaging methods with new molecular imaging probes and experimental therapeutic approaches targeting β-amyloid protein fibrillar aggregates were developed and tested in clinical trials. They were developed within a framework of the β-amyloid cascade hypothesis based on assumptions that β-amyloid protein aggregates, including fibrillar and oligomeric forms, appear as the initial pathologic event well before clinical symptoms of dementia become apparent.[1–4] Yet this hypothesis does not incorporate the effect of fibrillar hyperphosphorylated microtubule-associated protein tau aggregates commonly found in intracellular neurofibrillary tangles and neuropil threads, which, in addition to fibrillar β-amyloid protein aggregates found in extracellular β-amyloid plaques, are not only pathologic hallmarks of AD but required for definitive diagnosis of AD at postmortem histopathological examination.[5,6] From this perspective, the particular interest given to new imaging approaches using molecular imaging probes with ability to bind to brain neuropathologic insoluble protein deposits is not surprising. This new methodology could provide additional information about insoluble protein aggregate pathology in AD that is required for definitive diagnosis of AD and that was previously not available with imaging methods visualizing neurodegenerative changes on structural (magnetic resonance [MR] imaging) and functional ([F-18]FDG PET, measurements of perfusion with PET and SPECT methods) levels.[7]

Newly revised diagnostic criteria of preclinical AD,[8] of mild cognitive impairment (MCI) due to AD,[9] and of AD[10] now also include, for the first time, biomarkers of brain β-amyloid protein amyloidosis (cerebrospinal fluid [CSF] levels of β-amyloid proteins or PET imaging with "β-amyloid–specific" probes) and of neurodegeneration

Funding Sources: National Institutes of Health (P50 AG16570).

Conflict of Interest: None.

The author received support from the Mary S. Easton Center of Alzheimer's Disease Research at UCLA (NIH P50 AG16570).

Department of Molecular and Medical Pharmacology, David Geffen School of Medicine, University of California at Los Angeles, 10833 Le Conte Avenue, CHS B2-086B, Los Angeles, CA 90095-6948, USA

E-mail address: vkepe@mednet.ucla.edu

PET Clin 8 (2013) 431–445

http://dx.doi.org/10.1016/j.cpet.2013.08.002
1556-8598/13/$ – see front matter © 2013 Elsevier Inc. All rights reserved.

(CSF levels of hyperphosphorylated tau protein, atrophy measurements with MR imaging, and measurements of regional cerebral glucose utilization by using [F-18]FDG PET). As outlined in these guidelines, use of biomarkers of amyloidosis could potentially have an important role in early diagnosis of AD based on premortem detection of neuropathological deposits and could also bring new insights into the disease mechanism based on longitudinal monitoring of pathologic changes during disease progression, and significantly improve efficacy monitoring of novel therapeutic interventions focused on removal of insoluble protein deposits.

Based on this inclusion of PET imaging with "β-amyloid–specific" markers as one of the biomarkers of brain amyloidosis used for AD diagnosis, the Alzheimer's Association and the Society of Nuclear Medicine and Molecular Imaging have convened a group of experts to develop guidelines for appropriate use of "β-amyloid–specific" PET imaging.[11] The resulting criteria are listed in **Box 1** and they apply to several molecular imaging probes with claimed in vivo specificity for fibrillar aggregates of β-amyloid protein currently in use for human PET research in AD and related disorders: [C-11]PiB,[12] [F-18]flutemetamol,[13,14] [F-18]florbetapir,[15,16] [F-18]florbetaben,[17,18] [C-11]AZD2184,[19,20] and [F-18]AZD4694[21–23] (see **Box 2** for structures). Use of PET imaging with these "β-amyloid–specific" molecular imaging probes has also been reviewed extensively[24–40] from the perspective of their use as biomarkers of β-amyloid protein amyloidosis and, consequently, use of PET scans in diagnosis of AD, including early preclinical stages (eg, Refs.[24,25,27–33,35–37]), differential diagnosis (eg, Refs.[28,30,32,33]), for studies addressing mechanism of disease (as evidence for the β-amyloid cascade hypothesis [eg, Ref.[37]], longitudinal studies of disease progression [eg, Refs.[26,35,39]], correlations with other biomarkers, and tests of cognitive function [eg, Refs.[34,36]]), and finally to monitor efficacy of new therapeutic interventions aimed at reducing the β-amyloid aggregate load (immunization, gamma secretase inhibitors, and modulators) (eg, Refs.[24,41,42]).

But is the inclusion of PET imaging with "β-amyloid–specific" molecular imaging probes as biomarkers of brain β-amyloid protein amyloidosis warranted? Do we have unequivocal proof that PET signal accurately represents distribution and load of β-amyloid protein amyloid fibrils in a predictable and consistent way[43] to allow uses on the level of "proof of mechanism" and "proof of efficacy"[44] described in these articles? This article looks at some of these questions and, together

---

Box 1
Proposed use criteria

Amyloid imaging is *appropriate* in the situations listed here for individuals with all of the following characteristics:

Preamble: (1) a cognitive complaint with objectively confirmed impairment; (2) AD as a possible diagnosis, but when the diagnosis is uncertain after a comprehensive evaluation by a dementia expert; and (3) when knowledge of the presence or absence of Aβ pathology is expected to increase diagnostic certainty and alter management.

1. Patients with persistent or progressive unexplained MCI

2. Patients satisfying core clinical criteria for possible AD because of unclear clinical presentation, either an atypical clinical course or an etiologically mixed presentation

3. Patients with progressive dementia and atypically early age of onset (usually defined as 65 years or less in age)

Amyloid imaging is *inappropriate* in the following situations:

4. Patients with core clinical criteria for probable AD with typical age of onset

5. To determine dementia severity

6. Based solely on a positive family history of dementia or presence of apolipoprotein E (APOE)ε4

7. Patients with a cognitive complaint that is unconfirmed on clinical examination

8. In lieu of genotyping for suspected autosomal mutation carriers

9. In asymptomatic individuals

10. Nonmedical use (eg, legal, insurance coverage, or employment screening)

---

with a recent review,[45] raises questions about the interpretation of PET imaging data obtained with "β-amyloid–specific" probes.

PET SIGNAL AND MATCHING OF PET AND β-AMYLOID PROTEIN PLAQUE MAPS

Because β-amyloid protein fibrillar aggregates in β-amyloid plaques are the hypothetical target of "β-amyloid–specific" molecular imaging probes, PET imaging with these probes has to provide accurate quantitative in vivo information about β-amyloid plaque load in neocortical areas in complete agreement with postmortem determinations

Box 2
Structures of "β-amyloid–specific" PET molecular imaging probes

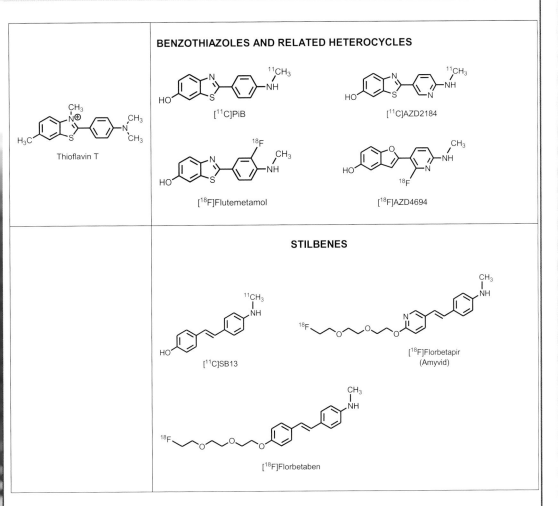

BENZOTHIAZOLES AND RELATED HETEROCYCLES

STILBENES

From Kepe V, Moghbel MC, Långström B, et al. Amyloid-β positron emission tomography imaging probes: a critical review. J Alzheimers Dis 2013;36:613–31; with permission.

of β-amyloid plaque load.[5,6] More specifically, recently updated National Institute of Aging/Alzheimer's Association (NIA/AA) guidelines for neuropathologic diagnosis of AD[5,6] require quantitation of β-amyloid plaque and hyperphosphorylated tau neurofibrillary tangle densities in a number of brain regions as a part of "ABC scores" determination:

1. A scores reflect stages of β-amyloid protein amyloidosis in structures of medial temporal lobe (MTL) as defined by Thal and colleagues[46,47] (see **Fig. 1** for depiction of these stages)
2. B scores are based on Braak NFT (neurofibrillary tangle) stages reflecting distribution of hyperphosphorylated tau protein fibrillar aggregates as neurofibrillary tangles and neuropil threads[48,49]
3. C scores are based on determination of cortical neuritic β-amyloid plaques in multiple brain areas as defined by Consortium to Establish a Registry for Alzheimer's Disease (CERAD)[50] (based on semiquantitative determination of senile plaque densities [sparse, moderate, frequent] in at least 5 neocortical regions, which must include the middle frontal gyrus, superior and middle temporal gyri, inferior parietal lobule, hippocampus, entorhinal cortex, and amygdala)

Because cortical β-amyloid protein amyloidosis is a progressive degenerative process, it follows a

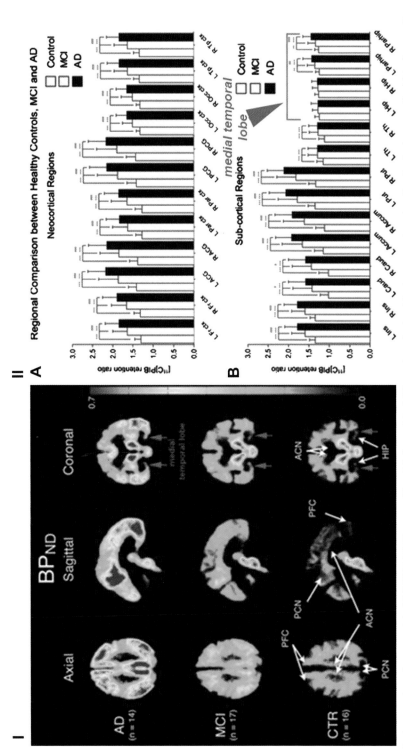

Fig. 1. Typical examples of parametric [C-11]PiB PET images (*Panel I*) from AD, MCI, and control subject groups showing the typical neocortical binding pattern with "silent" MTL structures. (*Panel II*) Results of quantitative analysis from a large [C-11]PiB PET multicenter study that are in agreement with the [C-11]PiB PET images shown in *panel I*. Panel IIA shows results for neocortical regions and panel IIB shows results for subcortical regions including limbic areas of MTL. Note apparent lack of [C-11]PiB binding in MTL structures in all subject groups. ([*Panel I*] *Adapted from* Devanand DP, Mikhno A, Pelton GH, et al. Pittsburgh compound B (11C-PIB) and fluorodeoxy-glucose (18 F-FDG) PET in patients with Alzheimer disease, mild cognitive impairment, and healthy controls. J Geriatr Psychiatry Neurol 2010;23:194; with permission.)

hierarchical order of regional brain deposition in the neocortex[48] and in structures of medial temporal lobe,[46,47] which are reflected in scores C and A, respectively. The initial deposits appear in neocortical structures of MTL, in inferior temporal lobe, and in orbitofrontal cortex (Braak amyloid stage A [see **Fig. 1**B] and Thal Phases 1 and 2 [see **Fig. 1**A]). From there, amyloidosis spreads to other neocortical regions (Braak amyloid stages B and C) and to limbic structures of MTL (Thal Aβ phases 3 and 4). Both directions of amyloidosis progression appear simultaneously. As shown in **Fig. 1**A//, Thal Aβ Phase 2 of MTL amyloidosis (dense amyloidosis only in neocortical structures of medial temporal lobe) occurs when Aβ deposition in neocortex is still limited to a number of isolated neocortical areas (Braak amyloid stage B). Patterns of cortical and MTL amyloidosis have also been described by other clinicopathological studies.[51–53]

Typical results of [C-11]PiB PET imaging in AD, MCI, and control (**Fig. 2**) subjects show distribution of elevated [C-11]PiB PET signal only in cortical regions of frontal lobe, parietal lobe with precuneus, and in lateral temporal lobe in patients with AD and in a subset of subjects with MCI[25,54] but not in the structures of MTL (including limbic and neocortical structures) in which the PET signal is unexpectedly low in all subject groups (see **Fig. 2**; **Fig. 3**). How can this be explained when β-amyloid protein amyloidosis in MTL structures is required for determination of the A score for AD diagnosis?[46,47]

This in vivo behavior of [C-11]PiB is incongruent with recently published in vitro results of [C-11]PiB autoradiography experiments performed with AD MTL tissue samples, which show robust [C-11]PiB binding in several areas paralleling the pattern of β-amyloid immunohistochemistry determined in these tissue samples[55] or the results of [H-3]PiB binding to AD brain tissue homogenates, which show high levels of [H-3]PiB binding in hippocampal samples.[56]

This unexplained in vivo behavior in MTL structures is not unique for [C-11]PiB, but is shared by all "β-amyloid–specific" molecular imaging probes, all of which appear to be "silent" in structures of MTL in vivo, even in the occipitotemporal gyrus (neocortical structure of MTL), which is one of brain regions with the earliest detectable β-amyloid aggregate deposition amyloidosis changes in the brain (see **Fig. 3**).[48]

VALIDATION STUDIES

A number of literature reports describe correlation of postmortem pathology with premortem PET imaging results with [C-11]PiB in AD,[57–60] in dementia with Lewy bodies (DLB),[61–63] in Creutzfeldt-Jakob disease (CJD),[64] and in Parkinson disease.[65] Two more articles reported results for [F-18]florbetapir.[66,67] None of them provides comprehensive analysis of MTL structures despite their unusual in vivo behavior in MTL structures.

Without rigorous validation, literature reports perpetuate unsupported interpretation of the observed lack of PET signal in MTL structures as resulting from the absence of β-amyloid pathology in all MTL structures in which tau NFTs are supposedly the prevalent type of pathology.[12,14,39] This interpretation is inconsistent with the NIA/AA guidelines for neuropathologic diagnosis of AD,[5,6] most specifically A scores reflecting β-amyloid protein amyloidosis in MTL. It has also been easily dismissed by immunohistochemistry (IHC) experiments using β-amyloid and tau antibodies on the whole-hemisphere tissue samples that provide information about relative densities of each IHC in MTL and other cortical areas (**Fig. 4**). This mapping methodology on whole-hemisphere tissue samples has been developed for determination of Braak NFT stages[49] but is equally useful for mapping of β-amyloid, as shown in a study describing mapping of pathology in a case of DLB[68] showing significant β-amyloid IHC densities in MTL structures (see **Fig. 4**).

The observed PET signal in brain cortical regions in AD and related neurodegenerative diseases is most commonly interpreted as resulting from binding of "β-amyloid–specific" probes to fibrillar Aβ, but conflicting results exist in the literature. In several publications, this correlation has been consistently established (eg, with total [both fibrillar and diffuse Aβ plaques] β-amyloid load[58] or only with diffuse β-amyloid plaques[62]). In other studies, only limited agreement of amyloid PET results with Aβ neuropathology (neuritic plaques measured using CERAD guidelines) are demonstrated with the investigators indicating that "…individuals with either intermediate or localized elevation of Aβ levels in vivo, variable agreement with diagnostic neuropathologic assessment was observed, even after applying several thresholds for positive scans (PiB+) and accounting for cerebral amyloid angiopathy (CAA)".[59] A significant number of studies report negative PET scan results in subjects with clinical symptoms of AD and cortical diffuse β-amyloid plaques (see, for example, Ref.[63]), which directly clashes with reports describing positive correlations between the presence of diffuse β-amyloid plaques and positive PET scans.[62]

A large number of cognitively healthy controls (~30%) show increased cortical PET signal, often

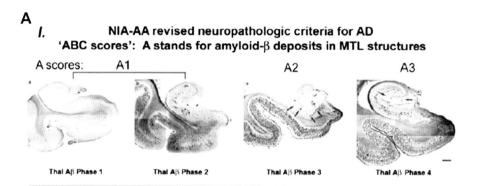

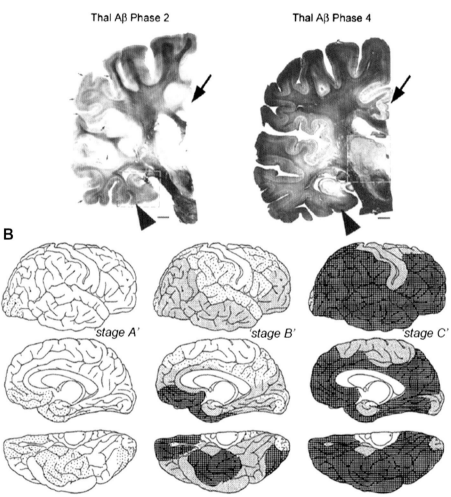

Fig. 2. Stages on β-amyloid protein amyloidosis in MTL structures (*AI-II*) and in the cortex (*B*). Both examples demonstrate progressive stepwise spread of β-amyloid protein deposition in both areas. AII: arrowheads point to MTL structures; arrows point to posterior cingulate gyrus. (*From* [*AI*] Thal DR, Rüb U, Schultz C, et al. Sequence of Abeta-protein deposition in the human medial temporal lobe. J Neuropathol Exp Neurol 2000;59:740, with permission; [*AII*] Thal DR, Rüb U, Orantes M, et al. Phases of A beta-deposition in the human brain and its relevance for the development of AD. Neurology 2002;58:1792, with permission; and [*B*] Braak H, Braak E. Neuropathological stageing of Alzheimer-related changes. Acta Neuropathol 1991;82:243; with permission.)

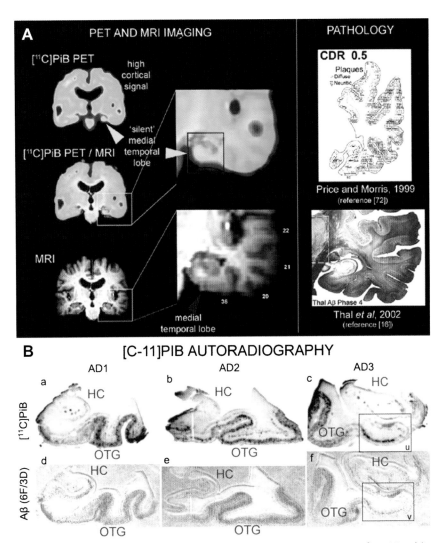

Fig. 3. [C-11]PiB PET does not show any appreciable in vivo signal in MTL structures of an AD subject despite the presence of β-amyloid aggregates (*A*). This is in stark contrast to the ability of [C-11]PiB autoradiography to label β-amyloid deposits in vitro in 3 MTL tissue samples from 3 patients with AD (*B*). Note good agreement between the [C-11]PiB autoradiography pattern and the areas labeled by β-amyloid IHC. ([*A*] *From* Kepe V, Moghbel MC, Långström B, et al. Amyloid-β positron emission tomography imaging probes: a critical review. J Alzheimers Dis 2013. doi:10.3233/JAD-130485, with permission; and [*B*] *Reproduced from* Harada R, Okamura N, Furumoto S, et al. Comparison of the binding characteristics of [18F]THK-523 and other amyloid imaging tracers to Alzheimer's disease pathology. Eur J Nucl Med Mol Imaging 2013;40:130; with permission.)

overlapping with the levels observed in patients with AD. Some patients with AD (~10%) show PET signal levels and patterns indistinguishable from controls (eg, Refs.[24,28,30,32]). Although these results have been interpreted as cases of preclinical AD in the control population, and as cases of dementias other than AD, as pointed out by Nelson and colleagues[69] in their recent extensive review of clinicopathologic correlation studies: (1) "it is extraordinarily rare for a case with widespread, dense AD-type neocortical lesions to lack documented *antemortem* cognitive decline" and (2)

"with some notable exceptions (eg, elderly schizophrenia patients, substance abusers, systemic disease), no significant subset of patients with severe age-associated cognitive decline exists that lacks any pathologic substrate when modern methods (ie, immunohistochemistry) are used in the neuropathologic examination."

Combined, these conflicting reports do not provide the expected validation of PET scans as biomarkers of brain amyloidosis, but rather raise additional questions about the true nature of the PET signal from these purported

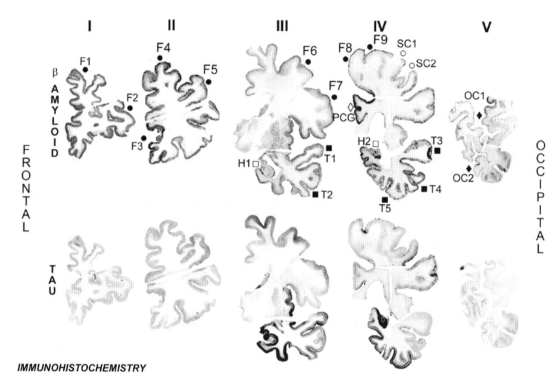

IMMUNOHISTOCHEMISTRY

Fig. 4. Examples of 3-dimensional mapping of β-amyloid IHC (*upper row*) and tau IHC (*lower row*) in brain tissue samples cut coronally at 5 levels from a hemisphere of a subject with DLB. Note medium to high densities of β-amyloid IHC in the MTL structures. (*From* Smid LM, Kepe V, Vinters HV, et al. Postmortem 3-D brain hemisphere cortical tau and amyloid-b pathology mapping and quantification as a validation method of neuropathology imaging. J Alzheimers Dis 2013;36:261–74; with permission.)

"amyloid-specific" imaging probes and their ability to accurately represent in vivo brain distribution and loads of β-amyloid fibrils in a predictable and consistent way.[43]

MOLECULAR IMAGING PROBE PROPERTIES

What is the reason for this variability? If we want to use PET with "β-amyloid–specific" molecular imaging probes for identification of subjects with preclinical AD as suggested by the guidelines for diagnosis of preclinical AD[8] or even for monitoring of anti-β-amyloid therapeutic interventions,[41,42] then we need to have clear understanding of the scope and limitations of this PET methodology.

The primary objective of PET imaging with molecular imaging probes in biomedical research is to provide quantitative information about dynamic physiologic processes targeted by these molecular imaging probes (eg, tissue perfusion, enzymatic synthetic processes, enzymatic metabolic processes, receptor related signaling) to assess changes between healthy and diseased states in living organisms, including human subjects.[43] Accurate quantitation and interpretation of PET

signal as an in vivo marker of the intended target is possible only if physiology of the process measured and biochemistry and pharmacology of the molecular imaging probe used are both properly characterized and included in a workable tracer kinetic model, and if the molecular imaging probe interacts specifically with the intended target. To meet these requirements, molecular imaging probes have to have a number of properties, summarized in **Box 3**,[43] including specificity of the molecular imaging probe for the intended target, low peripheral metabolism, and favorable transport between blood and tissue of interest, among others. Importance of these basic requirements for interpretation of imaging data was earlier highlighted by Dr Louis Sokoloff, a pioneer in the field of in vivo quantitation of glucose utilization with 2-deoxy-D-glucose derivatives, with a colorful example during his interview for the Archives of the American Academy of Neuropsychopharmacology in 2003 (available online at http://d.plnk.co/ACNP/50th/Transcripts/Louis%20Sokoloff%20by%20Thomas%20A.%20Ban.doc).

"… If one were to inject radioactive shoe-polish and image the radioactivity in the brain, one would

Box 3
Criteria for selection of molecular imaging probes for measurement of specific processes or organ function

1. Target specificity (ideally, the probe should be restricted to target process)

2. High membrane permeability to reach target areas

3. Trapping of the labeled molecule or labeled reaction product should occur in a slow turnover pool as a result of a specific interaction of target molecule (protein) in tissue

4. Use of analogs specific to one biochemical pathway to isolate one step or a few steps of the process; thus, the kinetics of only one administered compound is represented in the measured data

5. Rapid turnover rates (small precursor pool) for the substrate precursor are desirable to allow reaction of the labeled molecule probe to proceed rapidly and, thus, reduce background signal rapidly; this implies high affinity of the molecular probe for its target tissue and rapid clearance of the probe from nonspecific areas

6. Rapid blood pool clearance of the molecular imaging probe to reduce blood pool background at the tissue target (eg, brain, heart, tumor) and increase rate of clearance of the probe from tissue as a result of the temporal decrease in probe concentration in blood

7. No or slow peripheral metabolism of the probe to have the administered probe as the only or primary chemical entity in blood

8. High specific activity (low masses at the radioactivity concentrations used) to trace the process under investigation without exerting mass effect on the target molecule

9. Low nonspecific binding to increase target specificity and target–to–background ratios >>1

10. A small number of transport and biochemical reaction steps for the molecular imaging probe to allow tracer kinetic modeling to establish quantitative parameters for the imaging interpretation

almost certainly find patterns of distribution of radioactivity in the brain which might change with functional activation. One would not, however, obtain from the images alone any worthwhile information or useful knowledge about the nature of the processes involved that would allow one to design a model. Just injecting a radioactive compound

and getting an image is not enough. It must be combined with basic fundamental research beyond the imaging in order to get meaningful information. …"

Inconsistent results of PET imaging results with "β-amyloid–specific" probes and postmortem β-amyloid deposits require detailed reexamination of basic assumptions behind the PET data interpretation and further validation steps. If we fail to find plausible explanations based on experimental evidence, then basic assumptions need to be reexamined.

STRUCTURE-FUNCTION CONSIDERATIONS AND TARGET SPECIFICITY

The claim of in vivo specificity for β-amyloid protein aggregates with β-amyloid plaques was made first in the case of [C-11]PiB based on in vitro experimental results showing its ability to label to synthetic β-amyloid aggregates and human AD brain tissue homogenates, and its lack of ability to bind to other types of pathologic fibrillar protein aggregates (eg, tau protein neurofibrillary tangles, α-synuclein Lewy bodies) under the same experimental conditions.[12,70–73] These negative in vitro results with aggregates other than β-amyloid protein were interpreted as supportive of negative [C-11]PiB PET in neurodegenerative disorders associated with other amyloids, such as prion disease CJD,[64,74] synucleopathy Parkinson disease,[65] or tauopathies.[75,76] Other probes with similar PET imaging signal patterns in AD, MCI, and control groups than [C-11]PiB PET also bind to β-amyloid fibrils in vitro in the nanomolar range.[13,15,20,23]

Amyloid Structure

β-pleated sheet polymerization of misfolded soluble protein molecule monomers into β-pleated sheets[77–79] and their further association into protofibrils and rigid fibrils called amyloids, is characteristic of several brain proteins, including β-amyloid protein amyloid and hyperphosphorylated microtubule-associated tau protein in AD and Down syndrome, for prion protein in prion diseases, for α-synuclein found in Lewy bodies in Parkinson disease, and in DLB. Unbranched rigid fibrils of intermediate length formed by these proteins share common core properties,[78,79] that is, x-ray diffraction shows distinctive bands at approximately 4.8 Å and 10 to 11 Å, which are indicative of repetitive pattern of monomer's peptide backbone aggregated into β-pleated sheets via hydrogen bonds (4.8 Å band) and of stacking of multiple β-pleated sheets into protofibrils and fibrils (10–11 Å band). All types of amyloid fibrils are labeled by histologic dyes for amyloid fibrils (eg, Congo red, Thioflavins) and produce similar changes in spectroscopic properties of these dyes irrespective of the monomer protein structure.[78,79] Their binding ability must therefore depend on highly organized, repetitive nature of β-pleated sheets and rigid nature of fibrils present in all types of amyloid fibrils. These histologic dyes cannot be used to separate different types of amyloid fibrils (eg, separating β-amyloid fibrils from tau protein fibrils), which can be done only with IHC using antibodies raised against the specific monomer protein.

Although they are all invariably connected to human diseases called amyloidoses, amyloids do not possess any known physiologic function per se,[79] in contrast to physiologically active proteins (eg, receptors, enzymes, transporters), which have uniquely shaped spaces in their 3-dimensional structure that can accommodate their ligands or substrates with high specificity and affinity.[80] Successful PET molecular imaging probes for physiologically active protein targets are therefore often derived from chemical structures of the substrates/ligands or known agonists or antagonists of the specific protein function.[41] Based on their interaction with the active site(s) of these physiologically active proteins, their probes can achieve a high level of specificity for their protein targets and thus act as a biomarker of their protein target in healthy and diseased states of the organisms.[43]

Molecular Imaging Probe Structure and Properties

The "β-amyloid–specific" molecular imaging probes discussed in this article are based on 2 structural core elements:

1. 2-(4′-Aminophenyl)benzothiazole core element element: [C-11]PiB, [F-18]flutemetamol, and [C-11]AZD2184, as well as structurally related hydroxybenzofuran analog [F-18]AZD4694 (see **Box 2**)
2. Trans-stilbenes: the core trans-stilbene structure of [F-18]florbetapir ([F-18]AV-45) and [F-18]florbetaben ([F-18]AV-1) was claimed to be isosteric with the 2-(4′-aminophenyl)benzothiazole derivative [C-11]PiB,[81] which was then used to explain similarities found in in vivo PET scans and also similar binding affinities for in vitro formed β-amyloid fibrils

Based on of the ability of their parent compound (eg, Thioflavin T) to label all amyloids, one would expect that these probes possess similar properties. Curiously, claims of specificity for β-amyloid

fibrils are not based on structural properties of these imaging probes or those of amyloid fibrils. In vitro assays performed in solution with high alcohol content (eg, 10%), which strongly affect binding properties and do not mimic in vivo conditions, cannot be extrapolated to physiologic conditions in brain parenchyma.[12,13,15,20,23,70] Recently published [C-11]PiB binding experiments with in vitro–formed K18ΔK280-tau tau protein fibrils and with in vitro–formed Aβ42 protein fibrils in the presence of 0.2% bovine serum albumin in phosphate-buffered saline (instead of 10% ethanol) have yielded high binding affinity values to both types of fibrillar aggregates in the low nanomolar range: $K_d = 6.39 \pm 1.63$ nM for tau fibrils and $K_d = 0.84 \pm 0.18$ nM for Aβ42 fibrils, which contradict previous results in 10% ethanol (see previously in this article) and demonstrate the effect of experimental conditions in these in vitro determinations.[55]

Other factors that would significantly influence use of "β-amyloid–specific" molecular imaging probes as biomarkers of brain amyloidosis are (1) peripheral metabolism of probes forming metabolites that are capable of crossing the blood-brain barrier and accumulating in the brain, (2) metabolism of probes within the brain with consequent brain retention, and (3) presence of other, unidentified targets to which imaging probes could bind when present in the brain.[43]

From the perspective of signal interpretation, we need to consider that a PET scanner detects all radioactivity coming from the scanned tissue, for which the investigator does not have the ability of separating signal coming from different chemicals (eg, molecular imaging probe vs radioactive metabolites) or signal coming from molecular imaging probes bound to different protein targets, unless accurate biochemical correlates and models are rigorously established.

In vivo metabolism is a matter of concern for all probes with a free phenolic OH group in their structure ([C-11]PiB, [F-18]flutemetamol, [C-11]AZD1284, and [F-18]AZD4694). Phenolic compounds are prone to rapid and extensive conjugation via phase II metabolizing enzymes in the body[82]: for example, sulfation via sulfotransferases (SULTs), glucuronidation via uridine 5′-diphospho-glucurosyltransferase, and glutathione conjugation via glutathione S-transferase. Such conjugates can be trapped in the brain and cause radioactive signal unrelated to β-amyloid protein targets. Indeed, rapid peripheral metabolism of [C-11]PiB to its O-sulfate has been reported in rodents and humans,[83] although this radioactive metabolite is not capable of crossing the blood-brain barrier. But high reactivity of these

6-hydroxybenzothiazole probes with SULT enzymes increases the possibility of sulfation with SULT enzymes present within the brain,[84] as shown with the in vivo brain O-sulfation of [C-11] PiB in rat brain. Recent report of high-affinity estrogen SULT (SULT1E1) sulfation of PiB, flutemetamol, and other 6-hydroxybenzothiazoles (including 5-hydroxybenzofurans) raises significant questions about the nature of their in vivo brain signal in humans.[85]

Other unidentified brain targets binding [C-11] PiB have been recently reported in meningiomas in the absence of β-amyloid aggregates[86–88] and in [C-11]PiB PET scans of subjects with ischemic stroke[89,90] with increased level of [C-11]PiB binding in stroke-related neocortical regions. This points to the existence of brain cellular targets that are different from amyloids. In addition to these targets, [C-11]PiB has also been used for PET imaging of white matter changes in subjects with multiple sclerosis.[91]

Stilbene-based probes ([F-18]florbetapir, [F-18] florbetaben) also undergo rapid peripheral metabolism in humans to form a number of metabolites, including N-demethylated derivatives of [F-18]florbetapir[15,81] and [F-18]florbetaben,[92] which readily cross the blood-brain barrier, as demonstrated in rodent brains[15,81,93] and constitute approximately 44% of total activity in the rat brain at 2 minutes after intravenous injection.[93] These aminostilbenes are structurally similar to aminostilbene derivatives used as molecular imaging probes for in vivo visualization of myelin.[94,95] It is therefore not surprising that [F-18]florbetapir and [F-18]florbetaben PET scan results show a high degree of variability within each diagnostic group (AD, MCI, controls). Also in a recent [F-18]florbetaben study,[96] it was reported that "…images show a prominent signal in the white matter that contains no β-amyloid deposits. The exact cause of this peculiar high nonspecific binding of β-amyloid binding tracers in general is not known."

Interpretation of In Vivo PET Results

After considering all issues discussed up to this point about PET imaging with "β-amyloid–specific" molecular imaging probes, it becomes clear that multiple unresolved issues and lack of evidence for the claimed β-amyloid fibril specificity are detrimental to the interpretation of their PET signal as a measure of β-amyloid protein amyloidosis.

In the light of all questions raised, it is also worth noting that emerging data[97,98] point to discrepancies between results of [C-11]PiB PET studies and other imaging modalities (MR imaging, [F-18]

FDG) in cognitively normal elderly control subjects. In these subjects, the new guidelines for preclinical AD diagnosis propose use of PET imaging with "β-amyloid–specific" molecular imaging probes to detect brain amyloidosis as the initial pathologic event, as proposed by Jack and colleagues[99] in their new model of the AD pathologic cascade. Jack and colleagues,[97] as well as Wirth and colleagues,[98] have found a significant number of these subjects with negative [C-11]PiB PET scans but with abnormal MR imaging or [F-18]FDG PET measures, indicative of brain degeneration. This is in conflict with the proposed hypothetical model. Whether these observations point to the problems with β-amyloid cascade hypothesis (ie, β-amyloid aggregates are not initial pathology event) or to inability of these imaging probes to accurately reflect the presence of β-amyloid aggregates cannot be answered at the present time.

A recently published report by Roher and colleagues[100] further raises doubt about the ability of PET imaging with "β-amyloid–specific" molecular imaging probes to accurately measure changes in β-amyloid aggregate load resulting from therapeutic interventions: Rinne and colleagues[41] described an approximately 25% decline in [C-11]PiB PET signal levels in a group of patients with AD passively immunized with bapineuzumab, yet a follow-up postmortem pathology study in 3 patients with AD treated with bapineuzumab by Roher and colleagues[100] has shown no effect of treatment on histologically demonstrable leptomeningeal, cerebrovascular, and neuroparenchymal-amyloid aggregate densities in patients with AD treated with bapineuzumab when compared with a group of patients with AD used as a control in this study, which parallels findings on the lack of beneficial effects of these interventions on cognitive decline. Interestingly, no changes in CSF Aβ levels were observed in 69 subjects from the bapineuzumab study cohort,[101] but phosphorylated tau levels in the bapineuzumab group were decreased. In the words of Roher and colleagues[100]: "Coupled with the recognized complexity of AD biochemistry and neuropathology, these observations suggest that amyloid plaque deposits either cannot be the sole instigator of cognitive breakdown or their precise molecular constitution is of little overall consequence to dementia appearance. If this is the case, it suggests that despite remarkable impacts on AD biomarkers, the consistent lack of success of immunotherapy against dementia reflects the general failure to understand the function of amyloid deposition and its dynamics comprehensively."

This is not the first immunization study that failed to improve patient condition: Holmes and colleagues[102] reported follow-up results in 8 participants of the active immunization clinical trial with the synthetic Aβ42 peptide (AN1792) showing that among 8 subjects analyzed postmortem, 7 died in the stage of advanced dementia including 2 who had the highest titer of Aβ42 antibody and almost complete removal of β-amyloid from the brain. The investigators of this study pointed to the obvious lack of understanding between β-amyloid plaque deposition and cellular degeneration: "Our findings suggest that removal of Aβ plaques might not be sufficient to prevent the progressive neurodegeneration in Alzheimer's disease."

Continued speculations about the AD cascade and disease progression based on imaging results with purportedly "specific β-amyloid" PET molecular imaging probes, using questionable assumptions instead of scientific evidence puts us in no better position that the one described by Louis Sokoloff's example. The noncritical acceptance of the β-amyloid cascade theory based on "amyloid imaging" adds confusion to our understanding of the true nature of the mechanisms of neurodegeneration in AD and other neurodegenerative disorders.

Indeed, the lack of proper understanding of the true meaning of the PET signal obtained with "β-amyloid–specific" molecular imaging puts all of us in real danger of becoming prisoners of our own assumptions, similar to the prisoners in the Allegory of the Cave from Plato's *Republic,* who mistakenly take shadows and echoes for the real objects. In such situation, only proper scientific scrutiny and experimentation can lead to new insights and progress in the diagnosis and treatment of neurodegenerative diseases.

REFERENCES

1. Selkoe DJ. Alzheimer's disease: genotypes, phenotype, and treatments. Science 1997;275: 630–1.
2. Hardy J, Selkoe DJ. The amyloid hypothesis of Alzheimer's disease: progress and problems on the road to therapeutics. Science 2002;297:353–6.
3. Lambert MP, Barlow AK, Chromy BA, et al. Diffusible, nonfibrillar ligands derived from Abeta1–42 are potent central nervous system neurotoxins. Proc Natl Acad Sci U S A 1998;95:6448–53.
4. Lue LF, Kuo YM, Roher AE, et al. Soluble amyloid beta peptide concentration as a predictor of synaptic change in Alzheimer's disease. Am J Pathol 1999;155:853–62.
5. Hyman BT, Phelps CH, Beach TG, et al. Institute on Aging-Alzheimer's Association guidelines for the neuropathologic assessment of Alzheimer's disease. Alzheimers Dement 2012;8:1–13.
6. Montine TJ, Phelps CH, Beach TG, et al. National Institute on Aging-Alzheimer's Association guidelines for the neuropathologic assessment of Alzheimer's disease: a practical approach. Acta Neuropathol 2012;123:1–11.
7. Iqbal K, McLachlan DR, Winblad B, et al, editors. Alzheimer's disease: basic mechanisms, diagnosis, and therapeutic strategies. New York: Wiley; 1991.
8. Sperling RA, Aisen PS, Beckett LA, et al. Toward defining the preclinical stages of Alzheimer's disease: recommendations from the National Institute on Aging-Alzheimer's Association workgroups on diagnostic guidelines for Alzheimer's disease. Alzheimers Dement 2011;7:280–92.
9. Albert MS, DeKosky ST, Dickson D, et al. The diagnosis of mild cognitive impairment due to Alzheimer's disease: recommendations from the National Institute on Aging-Alzheimer's Association workgroups on diagnostic guidelines for Alzheimer's disease. Alzheimers Dement 2011;7:270–9.
10. McKhann GM, Knopman DS, Chertkow H, et al. The diagnosis of dementia due to Alzheimer's disease: recommendations from the National Institute on Aging-Alzheimer's Association workgroups on diagnostic guidelines for Alzheimer's disease. Alzheimers Dement 2011;7:263–9.
11. Johnson KA, Minoshima S, Bohnen NI, et al. Appropriate use criteria for amyloid PET: a report of the Amyloid Imaging Task Force, the Society of Nuclear Medicine and Molecular Imaging, and the Alzheimer's Association. J Nucl Med 2013;54: 476–90.
12. Klunk WE, Engler H, Nordberg A, et al. Imaging brain amyloid in Alzheimer's disease with Pittsburgh Compound-B. Ann Neurol 2004;55:306–19.
13. Nelissen N, Van Laere K, Thurfjell L, et al. Phase 1 study of the Pittsburgh compound B derivative 18F-flutemetamol in healthy volunteers and patients with probable Alzheimer disease. J Nucl Med 2009;50:1251–9.
14. Vandenberghe R, Van Laere K, Ivanoiu A, et al. 18F-flutemetamol amyloid imaging in Alzheimer disease and mild cognitive impairment: a phase 2 trial. Ann Neurol 2010;68:319–29.
15. Choi SR, Golding G, Zhuang Z, et al. Preclinical properties of 18F-AV-45: a PET agent for Abeta plaques in the brain. J Nucl Med 2009;50:1887–94.
16. Wong DF, Rosenberg PB, Zhou Y, et al. In vivo imaging of amyloid deposition in Alzheimer disease using the radioligand 18F-AV-45 (florbetapir F 18). J Nucl Med 2010;51:913–20.
17. Rowe CC, Ackerman U, Browne W, et al. Imaging of amyloid beta in Alzheimer's disease with 18F-BAY94-9172, a novel PET tracer: proof of mechanism. Lancet Neurol 2008;7:129–35.
18. Barthel H, Luthardt J, Becker G, et al. Individualized quantification of brain β-amyloid burden:

results of a proof of mechanism phase 0 florbeta-ben PET trial in patients with Alzheimer's disease and healthy controls. Eur J Nucl Med Mol Imaging 2011;38:1702–14.

19. Nyberg S, Jönhagen ME, Cselényi Z, et al. Detection of amyloid in Alzheimer's disease with positron emission tomography using [11C]AZD2184. Eur J Nucl Med Mol Imaging 2009;36:1859–63.

20. Johnson AE, Jeppsson F, Sandell J, et al. AZD2184: a radioligand for sensitive detection of beta-amyloid deposits. J Neurochem 2009;108:1177–86.

21. Cselényi Z, Jönhagen ME, Forsberg A, et al. Clinical validation of 18F-AZD4694, an amyloid-β-specific PET radioligand. J Nucl Med 2012;53:415–24.

22. Rowe CC, Pejoska S, Mulligan RS, et al. Head-to-head comparison of 11C-PiB and 18F-AZD4694 (NAV4694) for β-amyloid imaging in aging and dementia. J Nucl Med 2013;54:880–6.

23. Juréus A, Swahn BM, Sandell J, et al. Characterization of AZD4694, a novel fluorinated Abeta plaque neuroimaging PET radioligand. J Neurochem 2010; 114:784–94.

24. Nordberg A. Molecular imaging in Alzheimer's disease: new perspectives on biomarkers for early diagnosis and drug development. Alzheimers Res Ther 2011;3:34.

25. Nordberg A, Carter SF, Rinne J, et al. A European multicentre PET study of fibrillar amyloid in Alzheimer's disease. Eur J Nucl Med Mol Imaging 2013;40:104–14.

26. Resnick SM, Sojkova J. Amyloid imaging and memory change for prediction of cognitive impairment. Alzheimers Res Ther 2011;3:3.

27. Cohen AD, Rabinovici GD, Mathis CA, et al. Using Pittsburgh Compound B for in vivo PET imaging of fibrillar amyloid-beta. Adv Pharmacol 2012;64: 27–81.

28. Johnson KA, Fox NC, Sperling RA, et al. Brain imaging in Alzheimer disease. Cold Spring Harb Perspect Med 2012;2:a006213.

29. Klunk WE. Amyloid imaging as a biomarker for cerebral β-amyloidosis and risk prediction for Alzheimer dementia. Neurobiol Aging 2011; 32(Suppl 1):S20–36.

30. Villemagne VL, Rowe CC. Amyloid imaging. Int Psychogeriatr 2011;23(Suppl 2):S41–9.

31. Johnson KA, Sperling RA, Gidicsin CM, et al. Florbetapir (F18-AV-45) PET to assess amyloid burden in Alzheimer's disease dementia, mild cognitive impairment, and normal aging. Alzheimers Dement 2013. http://dx.doi.org/10.1016/j.jalz.2012.10.007.

32. Jagust WJ, Bandy D, Chen K, et al. The Alzheimer's Disease Neuroimaging Initiative positron emission tomography core. Alzheimers Dement 2010;6: 221–9.

33. Rowe CC, Ellis KA, Rimajova M, et al. Amyloid imaging results from the Australian Imaging, Biomarkers and Lifestyle (AIBL) study of aging. Neurobiol Aging 2010;31:1275–83.

34. Bateman RJ, Xiong C, Benzinger TL, et al. Clinical and biomarker changes in dominantly inherited Alzheimer's disease. N Engl J Med 2012;367: 795–804.

35. Gelosa G, Brooks DJ. The prognostic value of amyloid imaging. Eur J Nucl Med Mol Imaging 2012; 39:1207–19.

36. Pontecorvo MJ, Mintun MA. PET amyloid imaging as a tool for early diagnosis and identifying patients at risk for progression to Alzheimer's disease. Alzheimers Res Ther 2011;3:11.

37. Rabinovici GD, Jagust WJ. Amyloid imaging in aging and dementia: testing the amyloid hypothesis in vivo. Behav Neurol 2009;21:117–28.

38. Förster S, Yousefi BH, Wester HJ, et al. Quantitative longitudinal interrelationships between brain metabolism and amyloid deposition during a 2-year follow-up in patients with early Alzheimer's disease. Eur J Nucl Med Mol Imaging 2012;39:1927–36.

39. Mosconi L, Rinne JO, Tsui WH, et al. Amyloid and metabolic positron emission tomography imaging of cognitively normal adults with Alzheimer's parents. Neurobiol Aging 2013;34:22–34.

40. Villemagne VL, Burnham S, Bourgeat P, et al. Amyloid β deposition, neurodegeneration, and cognitive decline in sporadic Alzheimer's disease: a prospective cohort study. Lancet Neurol 2013;12: 357–67.

41. Rinne JO, Brooks DJ, Rossor MN, et al. 11C-PiB PET assessment of change in fibrillar amyloid-beta load in patients with Alzheimer's disease treated with bapineuzumab: a phase 2, double-blind, placebo-controlled, ascending-dose study. Lancet Neurol 2010;9:363–72.

42. Scheinin NM, Scheinin M, Rinne JO. Amyloid imaging as a surrogate marker in clinical trials in Alzheimer's disease. Q J Nucl Med Mol Imaging 2011;55:265–79.

43. Barrio JR. The molecular basis of disease. In: Phelps ME, editor. PET molecular imaging and its biological applications. New York: Springer; 2003. p. 270–320.

44. McCarthy TJ. The role of imaging in drug development. Q J Nucl Med Mol Imaging 2009;53(4): 382–6.

45. Kepe V, Moghbel MC, Långström B, et al. Amyloid-β positron emission tomography imaging probes: a critical review. J Alzheimers Dis 2013. http://dx.doi.org/10.3233/JAD-130485.

46. Thal DR, Rüb U, Schultz C, et al. Sequence of A beta-protein deposition in the human medial temporal lobe. J Neuropathol Exp Neurol 2000;59: 733–48.

47. Thal DR, Rüb U, Orantes M, et al. Phases of A beta-deposition in the human brain and its

relevance for the development of AD. Neurology 2002;58:1791–800.

48. Braak H, Braak E. Neuropathological staging of Alzheimer-related changes. Acta Neuropathol 1991;82:239–59.

49. Braak H, Alafuzoff I, Arzberger T, et al. Staging of Alzheimer disease-associated neurofibrillary pathology using paraffin sections and immunocytochemistry. Acta Neuropathol 2006;112:389–404.

50. Mirra SS, Heyman A, McKeel D, et al. The Consortium to Establish a Registry for Alzheimer's Disease (CERAD). Part II. Standardization of the neuropathologic assessment of Alzheimer's disease. Neurology 1991;41:479–86.

51. Arnold SE, Hyman BT, Flory J, et al. The topographical and neuroanatomical distribution of neurofibrillary tangles and neuritic plaques in the cerebral cortex of patients with Alzheimer's disease. Cereb Cortex 1991;1:103–16.

52. Price JL, Davis PB, Morris JC, et al. The distribution of tangles, plaques and related immunohistochemical markers in healthy aging and Alzheimer's disease. Neurobiol Aging 1991;12:295–312.

53. Price JL, Morris JC. Tangles and plaques in nondemented aging and "preclinical" Alzheimer's disease. Ann Neurol 1999;45:358–68.

54. Devanand DP, Mikhno A, Pelton GH, et al. Pittsburgh compound B (11C-PIB) and fluorodeoxyglucose (18 F-FDG) PET in patients with Alzheimer disease, mild cognitive impairment, and healthy controls. J Geriatr Psychiatry Neurol 2010;23:185–98.

55. Harada R, Okamura N, Furumoto S, et al. Comparison of the binding characteristics of [18F]THK-523 and other amyloid imaging tracers to Alzheimer's disease pathology. Eur J Nucl Med Mol Imaging 2013;40:125–32.

56. Niedowicz DM, Beckett TL, Matveev S, et al. Pittsburgh compound B and the postmortem diagnosis of Alzheimer disease. Ann Neurol 2012;72:564–70.

57. Ikonomovic MD, Klunk WE, Abrahamson EE, et al. Post-mortem correlates of in vivo PiB-PET amyloid imaging in a typical case of Alzheimer's disease. Brain 2008;131:1630–45.

58. Kadir A, Marutle A, Gonzalez D, et al. Positron emission tomography imaging and clinical progression in relation to molecular pathology in the first Pittsburgh Compound B positron emission tomography patient with Alzheimer's disease. Brain 2011;134:301–17.

59. Sojkova J, Driscoll I, Iacono D, et al. In vivo fibrillar beta-amyloid detected using [11C]PiB positron emission tomography and neuropathologic assessment in older adults. Arch Neurol 2011;68:232–40.

60. Driscoll I, Troncoso JC, Rudow G, et al. Correspondence between in vivo (11)C-PiB-PET amyloid imaging and postmortem, region-matched assessment of plaques. Acta Neuropathol 2012;124:823–31.

61. Bacskai BJ, Frosch MP, Freeman SH, et al. Molecular imaging with Pittsburgh Compound B confirmed at autopsy: a case report. Arch Neurol 2007;64:431–4.

62. Kantarci K, Yang C, Schneider JA, et al. Antemortem amyloid imaging and beta-amyloid pathology in a case with dementia with Lewy bodies. Neurobiol Aging 2012;33:878–85.

63. Ikonomovic MD, Abrahamson EE, Price JC, et al. Early AD pathology in a [C-11]PiB-negative case: a PiB-amyloid imaging, biochemical, and immunohistochemical study. Acta Neuropathol 2012;123:433–47.

64. Villemagne VL, McLean CA, Reardon K, et al. 11C-PiB PET studies in typical sporadic Creutzfeldt-Jakob disease. J Neurol Neurosurg Psychiatry 2009;80:998–1001.

65. Burack MA, Hartlein J, Flores HP, et al. In vivo amyloid imaging in autopsy-confirmed Parkinson disease with dementia. Neurology 2010;74:77–84.

66. Clark CM, Schneider JA, Bedell BJ, et al. Use of florbetapir-PET for imaging B-amyloid pathology. JAMA 2011;305:275–83.

67. Clark CM, Pontecorvo MJ, Beach TG, et al. Cerebral PET with florbetapir compared with neuropathology at autopsy for detection of neuritic amyloid-beta plaques: a prospective cohort study. Lancet Neurol 2012;11:669–78.

68. Smid LM, Kepe V, Vinters HV, et al. Postmortem 3-D brain hemisphere cortical tau and amyloid-β pathology mapping and quantification as a validation method of neuropathology imaging. J Alzheimers Dis 2013. http://dx.doi.org/10.3233/JAD-122434.

69. Nelson PT, Alafuzoff I, Bigio EH, et al. Correlation of Alzheimer disease neuropathologic changes with cognitive status: a review of the literature. J Neuropathol Exp Neurol 2012;71:362–81.

70. Klunk WE, Wang Y, Huang GF, et al. The binding of 2-(4'-methylaminophenyl)benzothiazole to postmortem brain homogenates is dominated by the amyloid component. J Neurosci 2003;23:2086–92.

71. Fodero-Tavoletti MT, Smith DP, McLean CA, et al. In vitro characterization of Pittsburgh Compound-B binding to Lewy bodies. J Neurosci 2007;27:10365–71.

72. Lockhart A, Lamb JR, Osredkar T, et al. PIB is a non-specific imaging marker of A peptide-related cerebral amyloidosis. Brain 2007;130:2607–15.

73. Fodero-Tavoletti MT, Brockschnieder D, Villemagne VL, et al. In vitro characterization of [18F]-florbetaben, an Aβ imaging radiotracer. Nucl Med Biol 2012;39:1042–8.

74. Hyare H, Ramlackhansingh A, Gelosa G, et al. 11C-PiB PET does not detect PrP-amyloid in prion

disease patients including variant Creutzfeldt-Jakob disease. J Neurol Neurosurg Psychiatry 2012;83:340–1.

75. Drzezga A, Grimmer T, Henriksen G, et al. Imaging of amyloid plaques and cerebral glucose metabolism in semantic dementia and Alzheimer's disease. Neuroimage 2008;39:619–33.

76. Tolboom N, Koedam EL, Schott JM, et al. Dementia mimicking Alzheimer's disease owing to a tau mutation: CSF and PET findings. Alzheimer Dis Assoc Disord 2010;24:303–7.

77. Eisenberg D, Jucker M. The amyloid state of proteins in human diseases. Cell 2012;148:1188–203.

78. Ridgley DM, Barone JR. Evolution of the amyloid fiber over multiple length scales. ACS Nano 2013;7:1006–15.

79. Stromer T, Serpell LC. Structure and morphology of the Alzheimer's amyloid fibril. Microsc Res Tech 2005;67:210–7.

80. Whitford D. Proteins: structure and function. Chichester (United Kingdom): Wiley; 2005.

81. Kung HF, Choi SR, Qu W, et al. 18F Stilbenes and styrylpyridines for PET imaging of Ab plaques in Alzheimer's disease: a miniperspective. J Med Chem 2010;53:933–41.

82. Kadlubar S, Kadlubar FF. Enzymatic basis of phase I and phase II drug metabolism. In: Pang KS, Rodrigues AD, Peter RM, editors. Enzyme- and transporter-based drug-drug interactions. New York: Springer; 2010. p. 3–25.

83. Mathis CA, Holt DP, Wang Y, et al. Species-dependent metabolism of the amyloid imaging agent [C-11]PIB. J Nucl Med 2004;45(Suppl):114P.

84. Miki Y, Nakata T, Suzuki T, et al. Systemic distribution of steroid sulfatase and estrogen sulfotransferase in human adult and fetal tissues. J Clin Endocrinol Metab 2002;87:5760–8.

85. Cole GB, Keum G, Liu J, et al. Specific estrogen sulfotransferase (SULT1E1) substrates and molecular imaging probe candidates. Proc Natl Acad Sci U S A 2010;107:6222–7.

86. Johnson G, Nathan M, Parisi J, et al. PiB PET/CT identification of meningiomas is not due to presence of amyloid-beta within tumors. J Nucl Med 2012;53(Suppl 1):253.

87. Bengel FM, Minoshima S. 2012 SNM Highlights Lectures. J Nucl Med 2012;53:15N–31N.

88. Kim HY, Kim J, Lee JH. Incidental finding of meningioma on C11-PIB PET. Clin Nucl Med 2012;37(2):e36–7.

89. Ly JV, Rowe CC, Villemagne VL, et al. Subacute ischemic stroke is associated with focal 11C PiB positron emission tomography retention but not with global neocortical Aβ deposition. Stroke 2012;43:1341–6.

90. Liebeskind DS, Kepe V, Cole GB, et al. PET of estrogen sulfotransferase in moyamoya syndrome: potential imaging of inflammation and arteriogenesis. Stroke 2011;42:E88–9.

91. Stankoff B, Freeman L, Aigrot MS, et al. Imaging central nervous system myelin by positron emission tomography in multiple sclerosis using [methyl-11C]-2-(4'-methylaminophenyl)-6-hydroxy-benzothiazole. Ann Neurol 2011;69:673–80.

92. Patt M, Schildan A, Barthel H, et al. Metabolite analysis of [^{18}F]Florbetaben (BAY 94-9172) in human subjects: a substudy within a proof of mechanism clinical trial. J Radioanal Nucl Chem 2010;284:557–62.

93. Jackson A, Smith GE, Brown SL, et al. Radiosynthesis, biodistribution and metabolic fate of three PET agents for amyloid-β in rats: [18F]flutemetamol, florbetapir F18 (18F-AV-45) and florbetaben (BAY 94–9172) (PW012). Eur J Nucl Med Mol Imaging 2011;38(Suppl 2):S231–2.

94. Wu C, Wei J, Tian D, et al. Molecular probes for imaging myelinated white matter in CNS. J Med Chem 2008;51:6682–8.

95. Wu C, Wang C, Popescu DC, et al. A novel PET marker for in vivo quantification of myelination. Bioorg Med Chem 2010;18:8592–9.

96. Becker BA, Ichise M, Barthel H, et al. PET quantification of ^{18}F-florbetaben binding to β-amyloid deposits in human brain. J Nucl Med 2013;54:730.

97. Jack CR Jr, Knopman DS, Weigand SD, et al. An operational approach to National Institute on Aging-Alzheimer's Association criteria for preclinical Alzheimer disease. Ann Neurol 2012;71:765–75.

98. Wirth M, Madison CM, Rabinovici GD, et al. Alzheimer's disease neurodegenerative biomarkers are associated with decreased cognitive function but not β-amyloid in cognitively normal older individuals. J Neurosci 2013;33:5553–63.

99. Jack CR Jr, Knopman DS, Jagust WJ, et al. Tracking pathophysiological processes in Alzheimer's disease: an updated hypothetical model of dynamic biomarkers. Lancet Neurol 2013;12:207–16.

100. Roher AE, Cribbs DH, Kim RC, et al. Bapineuzumab alters aβ composition: implications for the amyloid cascade hypothesis and anti-amyloid immunotherapy. PLoS One 2013;8:e59735. p. 16.

101. Blennow K, Zetterberg H, Rinne JO, et al. Effect of immunotherapy with bapineuzumab on cerebrospinal fluid biomarker levels in patients with mild to moderate Alzheimer disease. Arch Neurol 2012;69:1002–10.

102. Holmes C, Boche D, Wilkinson D, et al. Long term effects of Aβ42 immunization in Alzheimer's disease: immune response, plaque removal and clinical function. Lancet 2008;372:222.

Epidemiology and Clinical Diagnosis of Parkinson Disease

Michael Kleinman, DO*, Samuel Frank, MD

KEYWORDS

• Parkinson disease • Risk factors • Incidence • Prevalence • Diagnosis • Neuroimaging

KEY POINTS

- Parkinson disease (PD) is a common neurodegenerative condition.
- Numerous environmental factors are associated with either increased or decreased risk of developing PD.
- Incidence of PD has remained stable in recent years, although, because of an aging population, the number of people living with PD has been increasing.
- Diagnosis of PD is based on established clinical criteria based on pathologic data, but misdiagnosis is common because several related conditions have overlapping clinical features and lack of a clear biomarker.
- Neuroimaging can help confirm the diagnosis of PD in certain instances.

INTRODUCTION

James Parkinson[1] is credited as the first to describe the disease that came to bear his name in his classic "Essay on the Shaking Palsy," originally published in 1817. In this article he described the clinical features of 6 patients whom he thought had a disease that was yet to be characterized by neurologists. Although many genes have been identified as causing or contributing to the development of Parkinson disease (PD), most cases are considered idiopathic. PD is the second most common neurodegenerative disease behind Alzheimer disease and is the second most common movement disorder behind essential tremor (ET).[2] In addition to the disease burden, PD is the target of a major amount of government health care spending.[3]

RISK FACTORS

Age greater than 50 years and male gender are established risk factors for PD.[2] Men are 1.5 times more likely to develop PD than women.[4] There are several other risk factors that are less well understood and studied. Although no clear cause of PD is known, genetic susceptibility combined with environmental factors contribute to the risk of developing PD. A family history of parkinsonism, dementia, ET, and psychiatric disorder has been associated with an increased risk of developing PD.[5,6] In a recent meta-analysis, a family history of PD conferred the largest increase in risk of PD (odds ratio [OR], 4.45; 95% confidence interval [CI], 3.39–5.83).[6]

Other possible risk factors for development of PD include a history of pesticide exposure, head trauma, and heavy metal exposure (**Table 1**). The strongest example of chemical exposure causing a parkinsonian syndrome is the development of parkinsonism in drug users in California who inadvertently ingested 1-methyl-4-phenyl-1,2,3,6-tetrahydropyridine (MPTP).[7] Causality of drug ingestion for the development of parkinsonism in these patients was clear. There may be a risk of developing PD after exposures to other chemicals, but these relationships are less well established. Exposure to pesticides has been shown in a

Department of Neurology, Boston University School of Medicine, 72 East Concord Street, C-3, Boston, MA 02118, USA
* Corresponding author.
E-mail address: mkleinman@mmc.org

PET Clin 8 (2013) 447–458
http://dx.doi.org/10.1016/j.cpet.2013.08.005
1556-8598/13/$ – see front matter © 2013 Elsevier Inc. All rights reserved.

Table 1
Risk factors of PD

Established Risk Factors	Possible Risk Factors	Established Protective Factors	Possible Protective Factors
Male gender	Chemical exposure	Cigarette smoking	NSAID use
Age greater than 50 y	Heavy metal exposure	Caffeine consumption	Dihydropyridine calcium channel blocker use
Family history of PD	Head trauma	Increased serum uric acid	Alcohol use
—	Agricultural employment	—	Statin use
—	Well water drinking	—	Surgical menopause
—	β-Blocker use	—	—

Abbreviation: NSAID, nonsteroidal antiinflammatory drug.

meta-analysis to be related to the development of PD, with a summary risk ratio (sRR) of 1.62 (95% CI, 1.4, 1.88).[8] This analysis broke down the subtype of pesticides to herbicides, fungicides, and insecticides. Herbicides (sRR, 1.4; 95% CI, 1.08, 1.81) and insecticides (sRR, 1.5; 95% CI, 1.07,2.11) were associated with increased risk of PD, whereas fungicides (sRR, 0.99; 95% CI, 0.71,1.40) did not consistently show an increased risk of PD.[8] Likely related to chemical exposure, a history of employment in farming has been associated with a higher risk of PD.[6]

The association of head trauma with PD was first recognized among boxers in the 1960s.[9] However, the syndrome that these patients developed is not consistent with classic PD because cognitive dysfunction and psychiatric dysfunction were prominent symptoms, and this may have been the recently described entity chronic traumatic encephalopathy, a tau-related disorder.[10] The most recent and largest epidemiologic analysis of head trauma and PD showed that the strongest correlation between head injury and a diagnosis of PD was in patients who experienced a head injury within 1 year of a diagnosis of PD. For patients who experienced head injury up to 9 years before a diagnosis of PD there was a small but still statistically significant association. An increased risk of developing PD was not found in patients who were diagnosed with head trauma greater than 10 years before being diagnosed with PD.[11]

Long-term exposure to heavy metals has been hypothesized as a risk factor for PD. Exposure to high levels of manganese, such as in the mining industry, has been associated with the development of parkinsonism. However, a pooled analysis on the effect of manganese exposure did not show that this was associated with an increased risk of developing PD.[12] In addition to manganese, other heavy metals that have been studied in relation to

PD include iron, copper, and lead.[13–15] Results have been mixed for individual metals but chronic exposures to combinations of lead-copper, copper-iron, and iron-copper have been associated with an increased risk of PD.[13–15] One study found higher death rates caused by PD in counties with factories involved in paper production or industries related to chemicals, iron, or copper.[16]

The risk of PD caused by environmental factors is not always increased because some exposures reduce the risk of developing PD (see **Table 1**). The most robust associations have been shown for cigarette smoking and coffee consumption.[5,17–19] In a meta-analysis of caffeine exposure and risk of PD, caffeine consumption conferred a 25% reduction in risk of developing PD.[20] Most of the studies included in this analysis were restricted to coffee consumption. However, similar results are also seen for other sources of caffeine. Many studies have supported that smoking reduces the risk of PD, beyond the possibility of smokers dying earlier of other causes. A pooled analysis of epidemiologic studies of PD in the United States from 2007 confirmed the inverse relationship between smoking and risk of developing PD. The OR (95% CI) of developing PD among former smokers in the case control studies included in the analysis was 0.76 (0.68–0.86). The OR (95% CI) among current smokers in this group was 0.53 (0.44–0.63). The 3 cohort studies included in the analysis found an even greater risk reduction. In these studies the OR (95% CI) for former smokers was 0.64 (0.52–0.77) and 0.23 (0.15–0.36) for current smokers.[21] The protective association between smoking and PD has also been seen in people passively exposed to smoking. As in active and former smokers, a greater number of years of passive cigarette smoke exposure in the home is inversely related to risk of developing PD.[22] There is no difference ı mortality between patients with PD who were smokers versus never smokers. The mechanism or how cigarette smoking reduces risk of PD has ɣet to be established but may be related to mono-amine oxidase activity.

Increased serum uric acid levels have also been correlated with a reduced risk of PD, and patients with PD have lower uric acid levels compared with controls.[23–25] Patients with the highest quartile of uric acid levels in a population-based cohort study from 2005 had a hazard ratio (95% CI) for devel-oping PD of 0.42 (0.18–0.96).[23] In patients with PD, plasma uric acid levels were 13% lower than in controls.[25] The mechanism for how uric acid may reduce risk is speculated to be that uric acids function as an antioxidant and iron chelator. Increased iron has been found in the substantia nigra of patients with PD and increased iron may be associated with cellular damage related to oxidative stress and injury.[26]

The use of certain nonsteroidal antiinflammatory (NSAID) medications may reduce the risk of devel-oping PD. Although a meta-analysis found that overall use of NSAIDs does not reduce the rate of developing PD, when ibuprofen alone was stud-ed there was a significantly reduced risk of PD. This association was stronger for men.[27]

The use of dihydropyridine calcium channel blockers (DiCCBs) has been linked with lower rates of PD and a lower mortality in patients with PD.[28] In animal studies, DiCCBs alter the type of channels used by dopaminergic neurons for their pacemaking activities. As these neurons age, they switch from sodium channel activity to L-type calcium channel activity, which may make those neurons more prone to injury. Administration of DiCCBs switched the dopaminergic neurons back to using the more toxin-resistant sodium channel.[29] The hypothesis that DiCCB users are at a lower risk for PD is supported by the rates of PD in older patients (>65 years old) exposed to DiCCBs being lower than the risk of PD in patients less than 65 years old.[28]

INCIDENCE/PREVALENCE

Although methods and disease groups vary between studies, the incidence of PD and parkin-sonism consistently increases with age. In idio-pathic PD, there are issues related to the diagnostic accuracy because there is no clear biomarker for the disease. In the United States, the incidence of PD per 100,000 person years is 10.8.[30] In people 50 to 59 years old the incidence per 100,000 person years is 17.4. This number steadily increases to 93.1 in people who are 70 to 79 years old.[30] In a Canadian study, the

incidence in patients more than 65 years old was 252 per 100,000 person years.[31] A large European cohort study found the incidence of PD in people more than 65 years old to be 4.9 per 1000 person years.[32] In all of these studies the incidence of PD has been significantly higher in men than in women.

The number of people living with PD in the United States will increase in the coming years as the population ages. The 2005 estimate for the number of people in the United States with PD is 340,000.[33] By 2030 this number is estimated to grow to 610,000.[33] Worldwide, the largest in-crease in the number of people with PD will be in the developing Eastern nations, with a projected increase of greater than 100% in the number of people with PD in the most populous nations in the world (China, India).[33] A large European multi-national survey found that the overall prevalence of parkinsonism in people older than 65 years was 2.3 per 100 person years. The prevalence of PD was 1.6.[34] In Asia, the prevalence of PD in all age groups ranges from 51.3 to 176.9 per 100,000 person years.[35] In Africa, prevalence rates of PD are lower than in Western countries, ranging from 7 per 100,000 person years in Ethiopia to 43 per 100,000 person years in Tunisia.[36]

MORTALITY

Most studies of mortality in PD have shown higher mortalities than age-matched controls with reducing mortalities over the past few decades. The standardized mortality ratio (SMR) in people with PD in the prelevodopa era was reported as 3.0,[37] which is significantly higher than the results of more recent studies that have found SMRs of 1.1 to 1.77.[38–40] Some recent studies of patients with few significant comorbidities have found no significant increase in SMR.[41,42] Care in a special-ized movement disorders clinic has also been sug-gested as a factor in the wide variation of quality of care and SMRs in PD populations.

Time to death after a diagnosis of PD is highly variable. In a community-based study from Norway, the median survival time after motor onset of PD was 15.8 years, with a range of 2.2 to 36.6 years.[43] Mortality is similar among different worldwide geographic regions and within different regions in the United States.[44]

As expected, in addition to disease duration and severity, mortality is increased in patients with an older age at onset.[39,40] When examining disease severity with the Unified Parkinson's Disease Rating Scale (UPDRS), a 10-point increase in the UPDRS score was associated with a 40% increase in mortality.[45] When breaking down the motor score portion into individual items, worse scores for the postural instability and gait difficulty section are associated with increased mortality.[43] Other symptoms associated with increased mortality include the absence of rest tremor, symmetry of symptoms, dementia, hallucinations, and psychosis.[38,43,46–48] Factors associated with a faster time to the development of motor disability include the presence of levodopa-nonresponsive symptoms at the time of diagnosis, and cognitive dysfunction at the time of diagnosis.[49]

CLINICAL DIAGNOSIS

A diagnosis of PD should be considered in any individual who presents with tremor, bradykinesia, rigidity, or alteration in gait. Diagnostic accuracy is higher when considering the diagnosing physician's level of expertise. Diagnoses of PD by a specialized movement disorders service have shown a sensitivity of 91% and a positive predictive value of 98%.[50] Another study including diagnoses of PD made by general neurologists and geriatricians in addition to movement disorders specialists found that 76% of patients clinically diagnosed with PD had pathologic evidence of PD at autopsy.[51] A community-based study of the diagnostic accuracy of PD found that only 52% of patients diagnosed with presumed PD by general practitioners had clinically probable PD as assessed by a movement disorders specialist.[52] The cardinal clinical features of a patient presenting with early to moderate PD include rest tremor, bradykinesia, and rigidity. Although postural instability has been described as a cardinal feature of PD, this is typically a later feature of the disease and, if present early, may suggest an alternate diagnosis. There is currently no test that has proved to be specific for PD and therefore clinical criteria are relied on to make a diagnosis.

Physical examination of a patient being evaluated for PD should include a comprehensive neurologic examination to look for signs of parkinsonism, signs of atypical parkinsonism, and abnormalities that localize outside of the extrapyramidal motor system.

DIAGNOSTIC CRITERIA

There have been multiple attempts at developing diagnostic criteria for PD. The gold standard for a diagnosis of PD remains pathologic postmortem examination. Perhaps the most commonly used clinical diagnostic criteria are the UK Brain Bank Criteria (**Table 2**).[51]

More recently proposed guidelines break down diagnosis into definite, probable, and possible PD classifications. A diagnosis of definite PD requires histopathologic examination at autopsy. The diagnoses of possible and probable PD are based on the presence of a combination of the following findings: bradykinesia, resting tremor, rigidity, and asymmetric onset. Supporting features for diagnosis of PD include a documented clinical response to levodopa or a dopamine agonist, progression of symptoms, and the absence of exclusion criteria.[53]

Mental status testing is important to rule out significant cognitive dysfunction because this is not a feature typical of a patient with early PD. Dementia is significantly more common in PD than in the general population, with a prevalence rate among patients with PD of approximately 30%.[54] However, this aspect of disease is typically a late manifestation. Dementia, broadly defined, may be observed at the time of PD diagnosis in 8% to 16% of patients.[55,56] These numbers are skewed by changing diagnostic criteria for PD, inclusion of subcortical dementia, and by 35% of patients diagnosed after age 70 years already having signs of early dementia at the time of diagnosis.[56] The high association of dementia and PD in older patients has been attributed to the concurrent development of Alzheimer disease as well as a significant delay from the onset of motor symptoms to the time of diagnosis.

Bradykinesia

In the UK Brain Bank Criteria, bradykinesia must be present to make a clinical diagnosis of PD. Bradykinesia can manifest as reduced facial expression, slowed speech, slowed mental responsiveness, and slowness when performing motor tasks. The bradykinesia of PD is most often asymmetric and this is easily shown by observing for reduced arm swing when a patient is walking. Parkinsonian bradykinesia is distinguished from slowness of other causes by the reduced amplitude and speed of movements as well as the progressive slowness and reduction in amplitude when tasks are performed repeatedly. Bradykinesia in PD is caused by slowed motor planning, and slowed execution of movements.[57]

Tremor

The resting tremor of PD is viewed with the patient seated and the arms in a relaxed position. Tremor is most noted in the distal upper extremities and starts asymmetrically with an eventual spread to the contralateral side. The tremor frequency in PD is 4 to 6 Hz. The parkinsonian rest tremor of the hands is typically a pronation-supination movement giving it a pill-rolling appearance.

Table 2
UK Parkinson's Disease Society Brain Bank clinical diagnostic criteria

Step 1: Diagnosis of a parkinsonian syndrome	Step 2: Exclusion criteria for PD	Step 3: Supportive positive prospective criteria for PD • Three or more required for a definite diagnosis of PD in combination with step 1
Bradykinesia with at least 1 of the following: Muscular rigidity Rest tremor of 4–6 Hz Postural instability not caused by primary vestibular, cerebellar, visual, or proprioceptive dysfunction	History of repeated strokes with stepwise progression of parkinsonian symptoms History of repeated head injury History of definite encephalitis History of oculogyric crisis Neuroleptic treatment at onset of symptoms More than one affected relative Sustained remission Strictly unilateral features after 3 y Supranuclear gaze palsy Cerebellar signs Early severe autonomic involvement Early severe dementia with disturbances of memory, language, and praxis Babinski sign Presence of cerebral tumor or communicating hydrocephalus Negative response to large doses of levodopa in absence of malabsorption MPTP exposure	Unilateral onset Rest tremor present Progressive disorder Persistent asymmetry affecting side of onset most Excellent response to levodopa Severe levodopa-induced chorea Levodopa response for 5 y or more Clinical course of 10 y or more

Data from Hughes AJ, Daniel SE, Kilford L, et al. Accuracy of clinical diagnosis of idiopathic Parkinson's disease. A clinicopathological study of 100 cases. J Neurol Neurosurg Psychiatry 1992;55:181–4.

Postural and kinetic tremor also exists in PD, but to a lesser degree. Although tremor in PD usually starts in the distal upper extremities, it can also involve the lower extremities, jaw, and lips.[58] There are several key differences between the tremor of PD and the tremor of ET (**Table 3**). Despite these differences, a significant percentage of patients with PD are misdiagnosed as having ET.[59] A common pathophysiologic mechanism has been proposed because Lewy bodies have been seen on postmortem examination in brains of patients with ET and nigrostriatal dysfunction has been shown through imaging studies of patients with a clinical diagnosis of ET.[60,61]

Rigidity

Rigidity associated with PD is characterized by an increased resistance to range-of-motion testing throughout a joint's range of movement. Rigidity is a feature of PD in more than 90% of cases.[62] Rigidity can be shown in both proximal and distal

Table 3
Characteristic features of PD and ETs

Characteristic Features of Parkinsonian Tremor	Characteristic Features of ET
Most prominent at rest	Most prominent with action or sustained posture
Low frequency (4–6 Hz)	High frequency (7–12 Hz)
More likely to be asymmetric	More likely to be symmetric
Latency to onset of tremor with sustained posture	Absence of latency to tremor onset with sustained posture
Absence of head tremor	Head and vocal tremor may be present

joints and, like tremor and bradykinesia, is more likely to be asymmetric. Rigidity can be enhanced through the use of contralateral activation maneuvers.[63] Parkinsonian rigidity is described as cogwheeling, which is particularly apparent when an underlying tremor is present because this term derives from rigidity combined with tremor. However, cogwheel rigidity is not unique to PD because it is seen in many other neurodegenerative conditions as well as ET.

Bradykinesia and rigidity in a limb can lead to musculoskeletal pain, as seen in 33% of patients before a diagnosis of PD. The most common sites of musculoskeletal pain in PD include the back and shoulder.[64] Frozen shoulder has been seen in 12.7% of patients with PD. It is more likely to be seen early in the course of the disease and has been described as a presenting symptom of PD.[65]

Postural Instability

The loss of postural reflexes is generally a later manifestation of PD. Testing for abnormalities of postural reflexes is done by firmly pulling a patient backward from a standing position. If more than 2 steps are needed to maintain balance, or if balance would be lost without assistance, the test is considered positive. A decline in postural stability is a significant source of morbidity in patients with PD because of an increased frequency of falls. Meta-analysis of prospective studies of falls in PD has found that, in a 3-month period, falls occur in 46% of patients.[66] Other reasons for falls in PD include loss of proprioceptive input, muscle weakness, and a fear of falling that occurs after sustaining a fall.

In addition to the cardinal motor features of PD, there are several nonmotor symptoms associated with PD (**Box 1**). Some of these develop years before the onset of motor symptoms. Olfactory loss, constipation, and rapid eye movement (REM) sleep behavior disorder have been associated with a future clinical diagnosis of PD.[67–69]

RATING SCALES

The most common rating scale of disease severity in PD is the UPDRS, and more neurologists are moving toward using the updated version, the Movement Disorders Society-Unified Parkinson Disease Rating Scale (MDS-UPDRS).[70] The modified Hoehn and Yahr is the most commonly used PD clinical staging method (**Box 2**).[37,71] This scale has the advantage of ease of use and is also used frequently to characterize the disease severity of study populations.[72]

Box 1
Nonmotor symptoms of PD

Olfactory loss

Rapid eye movement sleep behavior disorder

Depression

Psychosis

Cognitive dysfunction

Pain

Sialorrhea

Autonomic nervous system dysfunction manifesting as:

    Orthostatic hypotension

    Constipation

    Urinary urgency/frequency

    Erectile dysfunction

    Temperature dysregulation

IMAGING

Advances in neuroimaging have allowed visualization of abnormalities in the midbrain as well as in the striatum in patients with PD. Magnetic resonance (MR) imaging, ultrasound, and single-photon emission computed tomography (SPECT) scanning have been extensively studied in PD. Although these technologies have shown promise as potential biomarkers for PD and can assist in making the diagnosis in certain cases, none of them have formally been incorporated into the diagnostic algorithm for PD. The key features of each modality in PD are summarized in **Table 4**.[73–78] MR imaging and SPECT in particular

---

Box 2
Modified Hoehn and Yahr scale

1.0: Unilateral involvement only

1.5: Unilateral and axial involvement

2.0: Bilateral involvement without impairment of balance

2.5: Mild bilateral disease with recovery on pull test

3.0: Mild to moderate bilateral disease; some postural instability; physically independent

4.0: Severely disabled; still able to walk or stand unassisted

5.0: Wheelchair bound or bedridden unless aided

Data from Hoehn MM, Yahr MD. Parkinsonism: onset, progression, and mortality. Neurology 1967;17(5):427.

Table 4
Neuroimaging in PD

Imaging Modality	Key Findings in PD
Susceptibility-weighted MR imaging	Increased iron deposition in the substantia nigra
High-field-strength MR imaging (7 T)	Irregularities in the lateral border of the substantia nigra Signal hypointensity in the dorsomedial aspect of the substantia nigra
Diffusion tensor MR imaging	Abnormalities in the diffusion of water along white matter tracts in the substantia nigra
Transcranial ultrasound	Increased echogenicity in the midbrain
SPECT scanning	Asymmetrically reduced dopamine transporter radioligand uptake in the striatum (putamen>caudate)

can be used clinically to exclude other diseases with parkinsonism based on clinical examination findings.

New MR imaging techniques have allowed the visualization of abnormalities in the substantia nigra of the midbrain. Studies of susceptibility-weighted imaging have shown iron deposition in the substantia nigra. The degree of iron deposition correlates with the severity of symptoms.[73] High-field-strength 7-T MR imaging has shown abnormalities in the lateral border of the substantia nigra with signal hypointensity in the dorsomedial aspect of the substantia nigra. These abnormalities corresponded with the side of the brain contralateral to the side of the body most affected by motor symptoms of PD.[74] Diffusion tensor imaging has shown abnormalities in the diffusion of water along white matter tracts using fractional anisotropy values in the substantia nigra of patients with PD.[75]

Transcranial ultrasound of the midbrain has shown an increased echogenicity in the substantia nigra of patients with PD. This finding has been seen in 9% of control subjects and 90% of patients with PD.[76–78] In a 5 year follow-up study, the degree of hyperechogenicity in the substantia nigra did not change as disease progressed.[78]

SPECT scanning has been used extensively to analyze the striatal dopaminergic system in PD and other parkinsonian disorders. The radioligands ^{123}I-β-carbomethoxy-3β-(4-iodophenyl) tropane (^{123}I-β-CIT) and ^{123}I-N-omega-fluoropropyl-2beta-carbomethoxy-3beta-(4-iodophenyl) nortropane ([^{123}I]-FP-CIT) both bind to the dopamine transporter, have been shown to have reduced uptake in the striatum of patients with PD, and have accurately differentiated between PD and ET in patients presenting with tremor.[79,80] [^{123}I]-FP-CIT is preferred for clinical use because it achieves peak binding in the striatum within hours after injection, whereas ^{123}I-β-CIT does not

achieve a stable level of binding for 14 to 24 hours.[81] A characteristic scan in PD shows asymmetrically reduced radioligand binding to the dopamine transporter in the striatum, with the putamen showing a more severe reduction than the caudate.[81]

PATHOLOGY

The gold standard for diagnosing PD is postmortem histologic examination of the brain. On histology, PD is characterized by a loss of dopaminergic neurons in the substantia nigra pars compacta of the midbrain as well as intranuclear cytoplasmic inclusions of the protein alpha-synuclein, which form Lewy bodies.[82,83] Lewy body features are also seen in structures outside the substantia nigra, such as the peripheral autonomic nervous system structures and cutaneous nerves.[84–86]

DIFFERENTIAL DIAGNOSIS

After it has been established that a patient has clinical features of parkinsonism, the next step is to determine the cause. A thorough medication history is important because numerous medications can cause a parkinsonian syndrome (**Table 5**), with neuroleptics causing the largest number of cases.[87] Misdiagnosis of drug-induced parkinsonism as PD is common, especially in the elderly population.[88] Diagnostic criteria for drug-induced parkinsonism include (1) the presence of 2 or more cardinal symptoms of parkinsonism, (2) absence of parkinsonian symptoms before exposure to the causative drug, (3) disappearance or significant improvement of parkinsonism after withdrawal of the causative drug, and no better explanation for the parkinsonism.[89] ^{1,2,3}I-FP-CIT SPECT scanning has been used to accurately distinguish between drug-induced parkinsonism and PD.[90]

Table 5
Medications associated with drug-induced parkinsonism

Class	Examples
Typical neuroleptics	Haloperidol, fluphenazine, thioridazine
Atypical neuroleptics	Olanzapine, aripiprazole, risperidone
Antiemetic agents	Prochlorperazine, metoclopramide, promethazine
Dopamine depleting agents	Tetrabenazine, reserpine
Other	Valproic acid

Cerebral vascular disease manifesting as a vascular parkinsonism (VP) is another common cause for parkinsonism. This diagnosis may be difficult to make because cerebral vascular disease is common in the elderly and may coexist with a diagnosis of PD. VP is more commonly associated with gait abnormalities along with non-motor symptoms including dementia, urinary symptoms, mood disorder, and sleep problems. VP rarely presents with rest tremor. Levodopa nonresponsiveness has been thought to be a component of VP; however, clinical improvement with low-dose levodopa has been found to occur in 77% of cases.[91]

Primary neurodegenerative diseases classified as atypical parkinsonism comprises the diagnoses of multiple systems atrophy (MSA), progressive supranuclear palsy, corticobasal degeneration (CBD), and dementia with Lewy bodies (DLB). MSA has subtypes marked by (1) prominence of parkinsonian features, (2) prominence of cerebellar features, (3) prominence of autonomic features. The subtypes of atypical parkinsonism can be differentiated from PD by several important clinical features (**Table 6**).[62,92–94] Common to all of the atypical parkinsonian syndromes is that they either do not respond to levodopa or the response to levodopa is not sustained.

CASE STUDIES
Case 1: Typical Idiopathic PD

A 55-year-old right-handed man with no significant medical history is seen because of right-sided slowness and changes in handwriting. He was first alerted of these symptoms 6 months earlier when a coworker commented that his right arm was swinging less than the left arm when walking. He had noted that his handwriting had become smaller and became progressively smaller and more difficult to read the more he wrote. He has also made more mistakes when typing over the last year. He has recent onset of mild aching of the right shoulder. He has not noted any changes in the left side of the body. He admits to some-times acting out his dreams over the past 5 to 10 years. He is on no medications and there is no family history of any neurologic disease.

Physical examination reveals a healthy-appearing man with normal facial expression and no mental status abnormalities. Eye movements are normal. There is mild rigidity with flexion/extension of the right wrist that is only present when he is asked to tap the left hand on his thigh. Repetitive finger and hand movements on the right side are mildly irregular and show decrementing amplitude with successive movements. Repetitive tapping of the right foot shows normal speed, rhythm, and amplitude of movement. Repetitive movements of the left side are also normal. Micrographia is evident when he writes a sentence.

Table 6
Atypical parkinsonian syndrome

Atypical Parkinsonian Syndrome	Differentiating Features from PD
MSA	
Autonomic predominant	Early severe autonomic dysfunction
Parkinsonian predominant	Poor and/or nonsustained response to levodopa, lack of rest tremor at onset, symmetric symptoms at onset, some degree of autonomic dysfunction
Cerebellar predominant	Prominence of cerebellar symptoms
Progressive supranuclear palsy	Presence of vertical gaze palsy Abnormalities of vertical saccades Falls within the first year of diagnosis
Corticobasal degeneration	Prominent and asymmetric dystonia, limb apraxia, and myoclonus
Diffuse Lewy body disease	Later age at onset, more prominent cognitive or psychiatric disturbances

There is no evidence of a rest, postural, or kinetic tremor. When walking he is noted to have reduced right arm swing without any slowing of walking or abnormalities of foot clearance or stride length. The patient's history and physical examination findings are typical for an early presentation of PD. In patients who present with bradykinesia and rigidity it is often the case that other people notice abnormalities before the patient does. Although his history of REM sleep behavior disorder predates his motor symptoms by several years, they are still likely related. In the absence of any features of atypical parkinsonism, further laboratory or radiologic testing is not likely to be of additional benefit.

Case 2: Drug-induced Parkinsonism

A 62-year-old man with a medical history significant for schizophrenia is referred for evaluation of 2 years of rest tremor. His medications include aripiprazole, lisinopril, simvastatin, and a multivitamin. On examination there is mildly reduced facial expression and blink rate. There is mild symmetric cogwheel rigidity of the upper extremities. Repetitive finger and hand movements are mildly slowed and with reduced amplitude on both sides. There is a 4-Hz to 6-Hz resting tremor in both hands at rest. A 1-cm to 3-cm kinetic and postural tremor is also present in the hands. There is an intermittent tremor of the lips as well. Strength and reflex examination is normal. His walking is slowed, with a stooped posture and bilaterally reduced arm swing. There is no postural instability. The differential diagnosis includes PD and medication-induced parkinsonism. A [123I]-FP-CIT SPECT is ordered to look for abnormalities of the striatal dopaminergic system. The scan shows symmetric radiotracer uptake in the striatum.

SUMMARY

PD is a common neurodegenerative condition that has a large impact on health care systems worldwide through increased morbidity and mortality. Although the exact cause of PD has yet to be elucidated, observations on environmental risk and protective factors for developing PD are providing clues to guide future research efforts. The diagnosis of PD is based on clinical grounds and is done without a high degree of certainty in many cases, because there are numerous illnesses that can seem similar to PD. The chances of arriving at a correct diagnosis of PD are increased through a careful history and physical examination along with the use of imaging modalities when indicated. The expertise of the diagnosing physician and the severity of the patient's symptoms increase the chances of arriving at a correct clinical diagnosis.

REFERENCES

1. Parkinson J. An essay on the shaking palsy. J Neuropsychiatry Clin Neurosci 2002;14:223–36.
2. Elbaz A, Moisan F. Update in the epidemiology of Parkinson's disease. Curr Opin Neurol 2008;21(4): 454–60.
3. Kaltenboeck A, Johnson SJ, Davis MR, et al. Direct costs and survival of Medicare beneficiaries with early and advanced Parkinson's disease. Parkinsonism Relat Disord 2012;18(4):321–6.
4. Wooten G, Currie L, Bovbjerg V. Are men at greater risk for Parkinson's disease than women? J Neurol Neurosurg Psychiatry 2004;75(4):637–9.
5. Savica R, Grossardt BR, Bower JH, et al. Risk factors for Parkinson's disease may differ in men and women: an exploratory study. Horm Behav 2013; 63(2):308–14.
6. Noyce AJ, Bestwick JP, Silveira-Moriyama L, et al. Meta-analysis of early nonmotor features and risk factors for Parkinson disease. Ann Neurol 2012; 72(6):893–901.
7. Langston JW, Ballard P, Tetrud JW II. Chronic Parkinsonism in humans due to a product of meperidine-analog synthesis. Science 1983; 219(4587):979–80.
8. van der Mark M, Brouwer M, Kromhout H, et al. Review is pesticide use related to Parkinson disease? Some clues to heterogeneity in study results. Environ Health Perspect 2012;340(3):340–7.
9. Lacava G. Boxer's encephalopathy. J Sports Med Phys Fitness 1963;168:87–92.
10. McKee AC, Cantu RC, Nowinski CJ, et al. Chronic traumatic encephalopathy in athletes: progressive tauopathy after repetitive head injury. J Neuropathol Exp Neurol 2009;68(7):709–35.
11. Fang F, Chen H, Feldman AL, et al. Head injury and Parkinson's disease: a population-based study. Mov Disord 2012;27(13):1632–5.
12. Mortimer JA, Borenstein AR, Nelson LM. Associations of welding and manganese exposure with Parkinson disease: review and meta-analysis. Neurology 2012;79(11):1174–80.
13. Weisskopf MG, Weuve J, Nie H, et al. Association of cumulative lead exposure with Parkinson's disease. Environ Health Perspect 2010;118(11): 1609–13.
14. Gorell JM, Johnson CC, Rybicki BA, et al. Occupational exposures to metals as risk factors for Parkinson's disease. Neurology 1997;48(3):650–8.
15. Gorell JM, Johnson CC, Rybicki BA, et al. Occupational exposure to manganese, copper, lead, iron, mercury and zinc and the risk of Parkinson's disease. Neurotoxicology 1999;20(2–3):239–47.

16. Rybicki BA, Johnson CC, Uman J, et al. Parkinson's disease mortality and the industrial use of heavy metals in Michigan. Mov Disord 1993;8(1):87–92.

17. Wirdefeldt K, Gatz M, Pawitan Y, et al. Risk and protective factors for Parkinson's disease: a study in Swedish twins. Ann Neurol 2005;57(1):27–33.

18. Checkoway H, Powers K, Smith-Weller T, et al. Parkinson's disease risks associated with cigarette smoking, alcohol consumption, and caffeine intake. Am J Epidemiol 2002;155(8):732–8.

19. Hernán MA, Takkouche B, Caamaño-Isorna F, et al. A meta-analysis of coffee drinking, cigarette smoking, and the risk of Parkinson's disease. Ann Neurol 2002;52(3):276–84.

20. Costa J, Lunet N, Santos C, et al. Caffeine exposure and the risk of Parkinson's disease: a systematic review and meta-analysis of observational studies. J Alzheimers Dis 2010;20(Suppl 1): S221–38.

21. Ritz B, Ascherio A, Checkoway H, et al. Pooled analysis of tobacco use and risk of Parkinson disease. Arch Neurol 2007;64(7):990–7. http://dx.doi.org/10.1001/archneur.64.7.990.

22. Searles Nielsen S, Gallagher LG, Lundin JI, et al. Environmental tobacco smoke and Parkinson's disease. Mov Disord 2012;27(2):293–6.

23. De Lau LM, Koudstaal PJ, Hofman A, et al. Serum uric acid levels and the risk of Parkinson disease. Ann Neurol 2005;58(5):797–800.

24. Davis JW, Grandinetti A, Waslien CJ, et al. Observations on serum uric acid levels and the risk of idiopathic Parkinson's disease. Am J Epidemiol 1996;144(5):480–4.

25. Annanmaki T, Muuronen A, Murros K. Low plasma uric acid level in Parkinson's disease. Mov Disord 2007;22(8):1133–7.

26. Mann VM, Cooper JM, Daniel SE, et al. Complex I, iron, and ferritin in Parkinson's disease substantia nigra. Ann Neurol 1994;36(6):876–81.

27. Samii A, Etminan M, Wiens MO, et al. NSAID use and the risk of Parkinson's disease: systematic review and meta-analysis of observational studies. Drugs Aging 2009;26(9):769–79.

28. Pasternak B, Svanström H, Nielsen NM, et al. Use of calcium channel blockers and Parkinson's disease. Am J Epidemiol 2012;175(7):627–35.

29. Chan CS, Guzman JN, Ilijic E, et al. "Rejuvenation" protects neurons in mouse models of Parkinson's disease. Nature 2007;447(7148):1081–6.

30. Bower JH, Maraganore DM, McDonnell SK, et al. Incidence and distribution of parkinsonism in Olmstead County, Minnesota, 1976-1990. Neurology 1999;52(6):1214–20.

31. Allyson Jones C, Wayne Martin WR, Wieler M, et al. Incidence and mortality of Parkinson's disease in older Canadians. Parkinsonism Relat Disord 2012;18(4):327–31.

32. De Lau LM, Giesbergen PC, De Rijk MC, et al. Incidence of parkinsonism and Parkinson disease in a general population: the Rotterdam Study. Neurology 2004;63(7):1240–4.

33. Dorsey ER, Constantinescu R, Thompson JP, et al. Projected number of people with Parkinson disease in the most populous nations, 2005 through 2030. Neurology 2007;68(5):384–6.

34. de Rijk MC, Tzourio C, Breteler MM, et al. Prevalence of parkinsonism and Parkinson's disease in Europe: the EUROPARKINSON collaborative study. J Neurol Neurosurg Psychiatry 1997;62:10–5.

35. Muangpaisan W, Hori H, Brayne C. Systematic review of the prevalence and incidence of Parkinson's disease in Asia. J Epidemiol 2009;19(6): 281–93.

36. Okubadejo NU, Bower JH, Rocca WA, et al. Parkinson's disease in Africa: a systematic review of epidemiologic and genetic studies. Mov Disord 2006;21(12):2150–6.

37. Hoehn MM, Yahr MD. Parkinsonism: onset, progression, and mortality. Neurology 1967;17(5): 427–42.

38. Herlofson K, Lie SA, Arsland D, et al. Mortality and Parkinson disease: a community based study. Neurology 2004;62(6):937–42.

39. Hely MA, Morris JG, Traficante R, et al. The Sydney multicentre study of Parkinson's disease: progression and mortality at 10 years. J Neurol Neurosurg Psychiatry 1999;67(3):300–7.

40. Auyeung M, Tsoi TH, Mok V, et al. Ten year survival and outcomes in a prospective cohort of new onset Chinese Parkinson's disease patients. J Neurol Neurosurg Psychiatry 2012;83:607–11.

41. Marras C, McDermott MP, Rochon PA, et al. Survival in Parkinson disease: thirteen-year follow-up of the DATATOP cohort. Neurology 2005;64(1): 87–93.

42. Montastruc JL, Desboeuf K, Lapeyre-Mestre M, et al. Long-term mortality results of the randomized controlled study comparing bromocriptine to which levodopa was later added with levodopa alone in previously untreated patients with Parkinson's disease. Mov Disord 2001;16(3): 511–4.

43. Forsaa EB, Larsen JP, Wentzel-Larsen T, et al. What predicts mortality in Parkinson disease?: a prospective population-based long-term study. Neurology 2010;75(14):1270–6.

44. Willis AW, Schootman M, Kung N, et al. Predictors of survival in patients with Parkinson disease. Arch Neurol 2012;69(5):1–7.

45. Vu TC, Nutt JG, Holford NH. Disease progress and response to treatment as predictors of survival, disability, cognitive impairment and depression in Parkinson's disease. Br J Clin Pharmacol 2012; 74(2):284–95.

46. Diem-Zangerl A, Seppi K, Wenning GK, et al. Mortality in Parkinson's disease: a 20-year follow-up study. Mov Disord 2009;24(6):819–25.

47. Lo RY, Tanner CM, Albers KB, et al. Clinical features in early Parkinson disease and survival. Arch Neurol 2009;66(11):1353–8.

48. Chen H, Zhang SM, Schwarzschild MA, et al. Survival of Parkinson's disease patients in a large prospective cohort of male health professionals. Mov Disord 2006;21(7):1002–7.

49. Velseboer DC, Broeders M, Post B, et al. Prognostic factors of motor impairment, disability, and quality of life in newly diagnosed PD. Neurology 2013;80(7):627–33.

50. Hughes AJ, Daniel SE, Ben-Shlomo Y, et al. The accuracy of diagnosis of parkinsonian syndromes in a specialist movement disorder service. Brain 2002; 125(Pt 4):861–70.

51. Hughes AJ, Daniel SE, Kilford L, et al. Accuracy of clinical diagnosis of idiopathic Parkinson's disease: a clinico-pathological study of 100 cases. J Neurol Neurosurg Psychiatry 1992;55(3):181–4.

52. Meara J, Bhowmick B, Hobson P. Accuracy of diagnosis in patients with presumed Parkinson's disease. Age Ageing 1999;28(2):99–102.

53. Gelb DJ, Oliver E, Gilman S. Diagnostic criteria for Parkinson disease. Arch Neurol 1999;56(1):33–9.

54. Aarsland D, Kurz MW. The epidemiology of dementia associated with Parkinson disease. J Neurol Sci 2010;20(3):633–9.

55. Foltynie T, Brayne CE, Robbins TW, et al. The cognitive ability of an incident cohort of Parkinson's patients in the UK. The CamPaIGN study. Brain 2004;127(Pt 3):550–60.

56. Reid W, Hely M, Morris J. A longitudinal of Parkinson's disease: clinical and neuropsychological correlates of dementia. J Clin Neurosci 1996; 3(4):327–33.

57. Berardelli A, Rothwell J, Thompson P, et al. Pathophysiology of bradykinesia in Parkinson's disease. Brain 2001;112:2131–46.

58. Jankovic J. Parkinson's disease: clinical features and diagnosis. J Neurol Neurosurg Psychiatry 2008;79(4):368–76.

59. Jain S, Lo SE, Louis ED. Common misdiagnosis of a common neurological disorder. Arch Neurol 2006;63:1100–4.

60. Louis ED, Honig LS, Vonsattel JP, et al. Essential tremor associated with focal nonnigral Lewy bodies: a clinicopathologic study. Arch Neurol 2005;62(6):1004–7.

61. Coria F, Gimenez-Garcia M, Samaranch L, et al. Nigrostriatal dopaminergic function in subjects with isolated action tremor. Parkinsonism Relat Disord 2012;18(1):49–53.

62. Louis ED, Klatka LA, Liu Y, et al. Comparison of extrapyramidal features in 31 pathologically confirmed cases of diffuse Lewy body disease and 34 pathologically confirmed cases of Parkinson's disease. Neurology 1997;48(2):376–80.

63. Powell D, Hanson N, Threlkeld AJ, et al. Enhancement of parkinsonian rigidity with contralateral hand activation. Clin Neurophysiol 2011;122(8): 1595–601.

64. Farnikova K, Krobot A, Kanovsky P. Musculoskeletal problems as an initial manifestation of Parkinson's disease: a retrospective study. J Neurol Sci 2012;319(1–2):102–4.

65. Riley D, Lang AE, Blair RD, et al. Frozen shoulder and other shoulder disturbances in Parkinson's disease. J Neurol Neurosurg Psychiatry 1989;52(1): 63–6.

66. Pickering RM, Grimbergen YA, Rigney U, et al. A meta-analysis of six prospective studies of falling in Parkinson's disease. Mov Disord 2007;22(13): 1892–900.

67. Ross GW, Petrovitch H, Abbott RD, et al. Association of olfactory dysfunction with risk for future Parkinson's disease. Ann Neurol 2008;63(2):167–73.

68. Abbott RD, Petrovitch H, White LR, et al. Frequency of bowel movements and the future risk of Parkinson's disease. Neurology 2001;57(3):456–62.

69. Iranzo A, Molinuevo JL, Santamaría J, et al. Rapid-eye-movement sleep behaviour disorder as an early marker for a neurodegenerative disorder: a descriptive study. Lancet Neurol 2006;5(7):572–7.

70. Goetz CG, Tilley BC, Shaftman SR, et al. Movement Disorder Society-sponsored revision of the Unified Parkinson's Disease Rating Scale (MDS-UPDRS): scale presentation and clinimetric testing results. Mov Disord 2008;23(15):2129–70.

71. Jankovic J, McDermott M, Carter J, et al. Variable expression of Parkinson's disease A base-line analysis of the DAT ATOP cohort. Neurology 1990; 40(10):1529–34.

72. Goetz CG, Poewe W, Rascol O, et al. Movement Disorder Society Task Force report on the Hoehn and Yahr staging scale: status and recommendations. Mov Disord 2004;19(9):1020–8.

73. Zhang J, Zhang Y, Wang J, et al. Characterizing iron deposition in Parkinson's disease using susceptibility-weighted imaging: an in vivo MR study. Brain Res 2010;1330:124–30.

74. Kwon DH, Kim JM, Oh SH, et al. Seven-Tesla magnetic resonance images of the substantia nigra in Parkinson disease. Ann Neurol 2012;71(2):267–77.

75. Cochrane CJ, Ebmeier KP. Diffusion tensor imaging in parkinsonian syndromes: a systematic review and meta-analysis. Neurology 2013;80(9): 857–64.

76. Becker G, Seufert J, Bogdahn U, et al. Degeneration of substantia nigra in chronic Parkinson's disease visualized by transcranial color-coded real-time sonography. Neurology 1995;45(1):182–4.

77. Berg D, Siefker C, Becker G. Echogenicity of the substantia nigra in Parkinson's disease and its relation to clinical findings. J Neurol 2001;248(8): 684–9.

78. Berg D, Merz B, Reiners K, et al. Five-year follow-up study of hyperechogenicity of the substantia nigra in Parkinson's disease. Mov Disord 2005;20(3): 383–5.

79. Asenbaum S, Pirker W, Angelberger P, et al. [123I]beta-CIT and SPECT in essential tremor and Parkinson's disease. J Neural Transm 1998; 105(10–12):1213–28.

80. Benamer TS, Patterson J, Grosset DG, et al. Accurate differentiation of parkinsonism and essential tremor using visual assessment of [123I]-FP-CIT SPECT imaging: the [123I]-FP-CIT study group. Mov Disord 2000;15(3):503–10.

81. Seibyl J, Marek K, Sheff K. Iodine-123-beta-CIT and iodine-123-FPCIT SPECT measurement of dopamine transporters in healthy subjects and Parkinson's patients. J Nucl Med 1998;39(9):1500–8.

82. Spillantini M, Schmidt M, Lee V. α-Synuclein in Lewy bodies. Nature 1997;388:839–40.

83. Spillantini M. Parkinson's disease, dementia with Lewy bodies and multiple system atrophy are α-synucleinopathies. Parkinsonism Relat Disord 1999;5(4):157–62.

84. Fumimura Y, Ikemura M, Saito Y, et al. Analysis of the adrenal gland is useful for evaluating pathology of the peripheral autonomic nervous system in Lewy body disease. J Neuropathol Exp Neurol 2007;66(5):354–62.

85. Ikemura M, Saito Y, Sengoku R, et al. Lewy body pathology involves cutaneous nerves. J Neuropathol Exp Neurol 2008;67(10):945–53.

86. Braak H, De Vos RA, Bohl J, et al. Gastric alpha-synuclein immunoreactive inclusions in Meissner's and Auerbach's plexuses in cases staged for Parkinson's disease-related brain pathology. Neurosci Lett 2006;396(1):67–72.

87. Bondon-Guitton E, Perez-Lloret S, Bagheri H, et al. Drug-induced parkinsonism: a review of 17 years' experience in a regional pharmacovigilance center in France. Mov Disord 2011;26(12): 2226–31.

88. Esper CD, Factor SA. Failure of recognition of drug-induced parkinsonism in the elderly. Mov Disord 2008;23(3):401–4.

89. Jiménez-Jiménez FJ, Ortí-Pareja M, Ayuso-Peralta L, et al. Drug-induced parkinsonism in a movement disorders unit: a four-year survey. Parkinsonism Relat Disord 1996;2(3):145–9.

90. Diaz-Corrales FJ, Sanz-Viedma S, Garcia-Solis D, et al. Clinical features and 123I-FP-CIT SPECT imaging in drug-induced parkinsonism and Parkinson's disease. Eur J Nucl Med Mol Imaging 2010; 37(3):556–64.

91. Glass PG, Lees AJ, Bacellar A, et al. The clinical features of pathologically confirmed vascular parkinsonism. J Neurol Neurosurg Psychiatry 2012;83(10):1027–9.

92. Colosimo C, Albanese A. Some specific clinical features differentiate multiple system atrophy (striatonigral variety) from Parkinson's disease. Arch Neurol 1995;52:294–8.

93. Respondek G, Roeber S, Kretzschmar H, et al. Accuracy of the National Institute for Neurological Disorders and Stroke/Society for Progressive Supranuclear Palsy and neuroprotection and natural history in Parkinson plus syndromes criteria for the diagnosis of progressive supranuclear palsy. Mov Disord 2013;28(4):504–9.

94. Stamelou M, Alonso-Canovas A, Bhatia KP. Dystonia in corticobasal degeneration: a review of the literature on 404 pathologically proven cases. Mov Disord 2012;27(6):696–702.

Dopamine Transporter SPECT Imaging in Parkinson Disease and Dementia

Devaki Shilpa Surasi, MD[a], Patrick J. Peller, MD[b],
Zsolt Szabo, MD[c], Gustavo Mercier, MD, PhD[d],
Rathan M. Subramaniam, MD, PhD, MPH[c],*

KEYWORDS

- Parkinson disease • Dopamine • SPECT • Dementia

KEY POINTS

- The diagnosis of Parkinson disease (PD) and dementia with Lewy bodies (DLB) is often not straightforward.
- When PD symptoms are atypical or overlap with other diseases (eg, essential tremor [ET] or drug induced), [^{123}I] N-ω-fluoropropyl-2β-carbomethoxy-3β-(4-iodophenyl) nortropane ([^{123}I]FP-CIT) single-photon emission computed tomography (SPECT) can improve the diagnostic accuracy.
- The potential side effects of medications for PD may be avoided, if [^{123}I]FP-CIT SPECT is normal. [^{123}I]FP-CIT SPECT is helpful in the diagnosis of DLB, differentiating it from other causes of dementia such as Alzheimer disease (AD).

INTRODUCTION

PD is a common neurodegenerative disorder characterized by progressive degeneration of dopaminergic neurons in the substantianigra, with loss of their nerve terminals in the basal ganglia structures, especially in the striatum.[1] The overall prevalence of PD is estimated at 0.2% but increases with increasing age, affecting as many as 0.5% to 1% of individuals aged 65 to 69 years and as many as 1% to 3% of individuals older than 80 years.[2]

PARKINSON DISEASE AND DOPAMINE TRANSPORTER SPECT

Parkinsonism is characterized clinically by deficits in motor function such as tremor, rigidity, bradykinesia (slowness of movement), hypokinesia (reduced movement), akinesia (loss of movement), and postural abnormalities.[3] The dopaminergic system is the most studied neurochemical system in patients with PD because damage to nigrostriatal neurons is the most important component in the pathophysiology of PD (**Fig. 1**).[4] The clinical diagnosis of PD is difficult, even by experienced neurologists, as several other neurodegenerative and basal ganglia disorders have similar clinical presentations. Overall, dopamine transporter (DAT) SPECT is most useful in discriminating between ET and parkinsonian syndrome with high sensitivity and specificity. It is also useful in discriminating between drug-induced parkinsonism (DIP) and degenerative parkinsonism because the former shows normal uptake. The most important management value is

[a] Department of Radiology, University of Alabama, Birmingham, AL 35249-6835, USA; [b] Department of Radiology, Mayo Clinic, Rochester, MN, USA; [c] Russel H Morgan Department of Radiology and Radiological Sciences, Johns Hopkins Medical Institutions, Baltimore, MD 21287, USA; [d] Department of Radiology, Boston University, Boston, MA-02118, USA
* Corresponding author. Division of Nuclear Medicine, Russel H Morgan Department of Radiology and Radiology Science, Johns Hopkins Medical Institutions, 601 North Caroline Street, JHOC 3235, Baltimore, MD 21287.
E-mail address: rsubram4@jhmi.edu

PET Clin 8 (2013) 459–467
http://dx.doi.org/10.1016/j.cpet.2013.08.006
1556-8598/13/$ – see front matter © 2013 Elsevier Inc. All rights reserved.

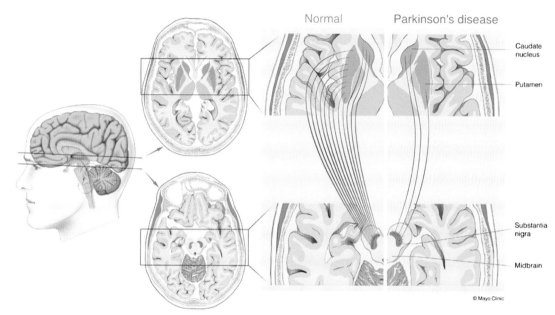

Normal   Parkinson's disease

Caudate nucleus

Putamen

Substantia nigra

Midbrain

© Mayo Clinic

Fig. 1. The main pathologic process in PD is nigrostriatal dopaminergic degeneration. The dopaminergic degeneration affects the putamen initially and then progresses to affect the caudate nucleus.

to exclude idiopathic PD as a cause of parkinsonian symptoms and thus avoid the long-term side effects from the anti-PD medications.

[123I]FP-CIT SPECT AND DOPAMINE TRANSPORTER

The active ingredient of [123I]FP-CIT SPECT is a cocaine analogue, 123I-labeled *N*-ω-fluoropropyl 2β-carbomethoxy-3β-(4-iodophenyl) nortropane ([123I]ioflupane). It binds with high affinity to striatal presynaptic DAT in animals and in humans[5] and helps visualize these neurons with SPECT brain imaging. [123I]FP-CIT SPECT has the advantage of faster kinetics, which allows imaging 3 to 6 hours after injection. [123I]FP-CIT is currently classified as a controlled substance (Schedule II) drug under the Controlled Substances Act in the United States, as the imaging agent is related to the active ingredient in cocaine. Thus, in the United States, an authorized user of radiopharmaceuticals must also have a narcotic license (Drug Enforcement Administration license) to order and administer the agent.[6]

DAT is located on the plasma membrane of nerve terminals in a small number of neurons in the brain, especially in the striatum and nucleus accumbens, and in the globus pallidus, cingulate cortex, olfactory tubercle, amygdala, and midbrain.[7] DAT regulates the dopamine concentration in the synaptic cleft through reuptake of dopamine into presynaptic neurons and thus plays a central role in the buffering of the released dopamine (**Fig. 2**).[8]

[123I]FP-CIT SPECT IMAGING PROTOCOL

Patient preparation: Patients should increase the intake of fluids because the tracer is excreted largely in the urine. After injection, the fluid intake

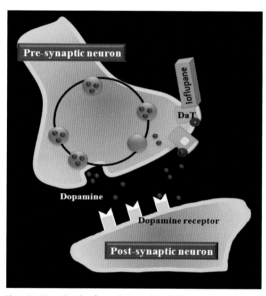

Fig. 2. Terminal of a nigrostriatal dopaminergic cell and a postsynaptic cell. Dopamine synthesized in the dopaminergic neurons is stored in the vesicle, is released in response to an action potential into the synaptic cleft, and interacts with the dopamine receptors. The extracellular dopamine is actively pumped back into the dopaminergic terminal by the dopaminergic transporter (DaT). Ioflupane binds to DaT on the nigrostriatal neurons.

should continue, with increased frequency of voiding for the next 48 hours. The preparation has a significant fraction of free iodine 123 (up to 6%), which accumulates in the thyroid gland. Patients must thus be pretreated to block the uptake of radioactive iodine into the thyroid gland by the administration of saturated solution of potassium iodide or Lugol solution. Renal or hepatic dysfunction may impair the excretion of the tracer. History of allergic reaction to [123I]FP-CIT or iodine must be ruled out, but allergy to FP-CIT is not well established and allergy to iodine is rare. It should be used in pregnant women only when clearly indicated and all diagnostic evaluations are equivocal. Nursing mothers may receive the tracer, but breast milk should be discarded for at least 6 days to avoid radiation exposure of the infant.

The dose for adults is 5 mCi (185 MBq), injected intravenously. Time from injection to start of data acquisition is 3 to 6 hours after injection for [123I]ioflupane. The patient must be encouraged to void before the scan and placed in a supine comfortable position. Multiple detector (triple or dual head) or other dedicated SPECT cameras for brain imaging should be used for data acquisition.[9] The patient's head must be maintained symmetric during the scan. Asymmetric position of the head can be corrected by image rotation, but it may still lead to overinterpretation of the scan and increased rate of false-positive results. Acquisition parameters include the smallest possible rotational radius 11 to 13 cm, 128 × 128 matrix, and angular sampling of 3° (360° rotation). Acquisition pixel size should be one-third to one-half of the expected resolution; therefore, it may be necessary to use a hardware zoom to achieve an appropriate pixel size. For acquisition mode, step and shoot mode is used predominantly. Continuous mode acquisition may provide shorter total scan times and reduce mechanical wear to the system. The total detected events include greater than 1.5 million counts. When iterative reconstruction with scatter correction is applied, lower numbers may be acceptable. The total scan time for a triple-head camera is around 30 min (eg, 120 projections; 40 projections per head; 45 seconds per projection). Segmentation of data acquisition into multiple sequential acquisitions may permit exclusion of data with artifacts, for example, remove segments of projection data with patient motion.[10] Images may be reconstructed using either a filter back projection or an iterative reconstruction algorithm. For attenuation correction, an attenuation map is acquired with an external source or computed tomography. A simplified technique of attenuation correction is based on a map obtained with the Chang algorithm.

There are certain drugs that may interfere with [123I]FP-CIT SPECT (**Table 1**). The use of these medications need to be stopped (ideally 6 T1/2s) before the scan. Selective serotonin reuptake inhibitors such as paroxetine and citalopram interfere with quantification but not visual interpretation. Cholinesterase inhibitors and antiparkinsonian drugs such as L-dopa, amantidine, catechol-O-methyl transferase inhibitors, monoamine oxidase B inhibitors, N-methyl-D-aspartate receptor blockers, and dopamine agonists are unlikely to interfere with the scan.[10,11]

[123I]FP-CIT SPECT INTERPRETATION

Interpretation is done either through computer-aided quantification or by qualitative reading of uptake in the striatum. In the United States, Food and Drug Administration approval of the tracer is based on qualitative reading against a standard atlas composed of images. Normal distribution is a comma-shaped area of uptake in the striatum that includes the caudate and putamen. This uptake is intense with little background in the remainder of the brain and symmetric without left-to-right or anterior-to-posterior gradients (**Fig. 3**).

Abnormal uptake takes several patterns. Traditional PD demonstrates decreased activity in the putamen, worse on the side contralateral to dominant motor symptoms. With progression of disease, the deficit spreads to both sides and then to the

Table 1 Effects of drugs	
Decrease Striatal Binding	**Increase Striatal Binding**
Cocaine	Adrenergic agonists (phenylephrine, norepinephrine)
Amphetamines (D-amphetamine, methamphetamine, methylphenidate)	Anticholinergics
CNS stimulants (phentermine, ephedrines)	
Modafinil	
Antidepressants (mazindol, bupropion, radafaxine)	
Opioids, fentanyl	
Anesthetics (ketamine, PCP, isoflurane)	

Abbreviations: CNS, central nervous system; PCP, phencyclidine.

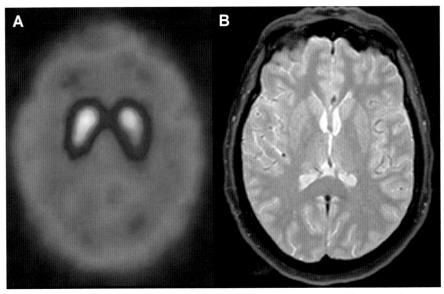

Fig. 3. [^{123}I]FP-CIT SPECT—normal scan result. (*A*) [^{123}I]FP-CIT SPECT in a 63-year-old woman demonstrates signal in the striata. Bilateral crescent shapes consistent with normal dopaminergic neurons. (*B*) Axial sT2/PD MR imaging demonstrates normal anatomy of the striata and no other significant abnormalities.

caudate nucleus. **Fig. 4** shows progressive loss of the DAT consistent with presynaptic neuronal loss in the striatum. The result is a change from a bilateral "comma" to dots that represent residual uptake in the caudate nucleus. With increasing disease severity, uptake is further reduced so that background uptake becomes more evident. One caveat in qualitative interpretation is the need for rigorous attention to symmetric orientation of the brain and no motion during imaging. It may be necessary to perform oblique reconstructions to correct for patient position, but the scan may have to be repeated in the event of significant motion.

The quantification of [^{123}I]FP-CIT SPECT images are at an investigational stage and can be done using software program to assess the uptake in the striatum. QuantiSPECT (GE Healthcare, WI, USA) processes the data in 2 dimensions, and BRASS (brain reorientation and analysis, HERMES Medical Solutions, Stockholm, Sweden) program processes in 3 dimensions. Mortan and colleagues[12] compared these 2 programs, assessing the intrareader and interreader variation. A 3% intraoperator variability was found using BRASS program, and the variability using QuantiSPECT ranged from 4% to 8%.[12]

DIAGNOSIS

The interval between the onset of loss of nigral dopaminergic neurons and the onset of clinical symptoms of PD is unknown. Fearnley and Lees[13] calculated a preclinical window of around

6 years based on the findings of exponential rates of nigral cell loss in a postmortem series of brains of patients with PD. The first motor symptoms of PD occur after 80% of striatal and 50% of nigral dopamine cells are lost.

Dopamine SPECT is valuable in early diagnosis of idiopathic PD. Marek and colleagues[14] studied SPECT with [^{123}I] beta-CIT to investigate striatal DAT loss in patients with early PD. They compared striatal uptake of [^{123}I] beta-CIT in 8 patients with early-PD with hemiparkinsonism and 8 age- and sex-matched healthy subjects and found that the striatal uptake was reduced by approximately 53% contralateral and 38% ipsilateral to the clinically symptomatic side in the patients with hemi-PD, compared with the mean striatal uptake in age- and sex-matched healthy subjects, thus demonstrating that SPECT imaging of the DAT with [^{123}I] beta-CIT can identify patients with PD at the onset of motor symptoms.

A meta-analysis was conducted by Vlaar and colleagues[15] to review the diagnostic accuracy of SPECT to differentiate between early phase of PD and normalcy. All the 6 cross-sectional studies (using presynaptic tracers) with patients with known PD in an early stage (Hoehn and Yahr score of 2 or lesser) had a specificity of 100% and the sensitivity varied from 8% to 100%.[15] The details of the 6 studies are elaborated in **Table 2**.[16–21] Diagnosis of PD in the early stages of the disease is necessary for the appropriate management. Recent studies such as [TVP-1012] in Early Monotherapy for Parkinson's disease Outpatients (TEMPO) and Earlier

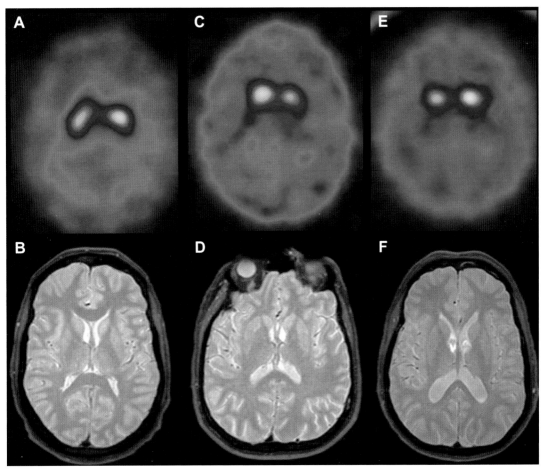

Fig. 4. [^{123}I]FP-CIT SPECT—abnormal scan results. (*A, B*) [^{123}I]FP-CIT SPECT demonstrates decreased signal asymmetrically. There is greater reduction in the left striatum than in the right. Axial sT2/PD MR imaging demonstrates normal anatomy of the striata and no other significant abnormalities. (*C, D*) [^{123}I]FP-CIT SPECT demonstrates decreased signal asymmetrically on both striata and asymmetrically decreased signal in the left caudate nucleus. Axial sT2/PD MR imaging demonstrates normal anatomy of the striata and no other significant abnormalities. (*E, F*) [^{123}I]FP-CIT SPECT demonstrates decreased signal bilaterally and almost symmetrically. Axial sT2/PD MR imaging demonstrates normal anatomy of the striata and no other significant abnormalities.

versus Later Levodopa Therapy in Parkinson's Disease (ELLDOPA) suggest that early treatment may provide a better outcome than a delayed one.[22,23] Dopamine SPECT shows a progressive decline of striatal DAT binding with the duration of PD and with increasing disease severity and thus has been used as a potential biomarker for disease progression in PD.[24]

Table 2
Diagnostic accuracy of SPECT in differentiating patients with early PD and normal subjects

Author	PD (*n*)	Controls (*n*)	TP	FN	TN	FP	Sensitivity	Specificity	Odds Ratio
Asenbaum et al,[16] 1998	29	30	23	6	30	0	79	100	235
Haapaniemi et al,[17] 2001	29	21	16	13	21	0	55	100	52
Huang et al,[18] 2001	34	17	32	2	17	0	94	100	455
Muller et al,[19] 1998	24	15	14	10	15	0	58	100	42
Schwarz et al,[20] 2000	28	9	28	0	9	0	100	100	1083
Van Laere et al,[21] 2004	39	10	15	24	10	0	38	100	13

Abbreviations: FN, false negative; FP, false positive; TN, true negative; TP, true positives.

ASSESSMENT OF PROGRESSION OF DISEASE

Dopamine SPECT studies may be helpful in the assessment of progression of PD. In a longitudinal study assessing PD progression, the annual rate of reduction of striatal DAT uptake was approximately 6% to 13% in PD patients, compared with 0% to 2.5% in healthy controls, which was in line with the results from [18F] dopa-PET studies.[25–27] The percentage of change from baseline of striatal dopamine SPECT has been used as an index for disease progression in several clinical trials with levodopa, selegiline, and pramipexole.[23,28] There is an ongoing international multicenter longitudinal study—Parkinson's Progressive Markers Initiative—with [123I]FP-CIT SPECT, MR imaging, and other biologic markers.[29]

TREATMENT MONITORING

Dopamine SPECT has been used for treatment monitoring trials in PD. Several landmark trials have been described investigating the early treatment of PD.[30] The Parkinson study group conducted a randomized clinical trial involving a subgroup of 82 early patients with PD who were randomized 1:1 to the dopamine agonist pramipexole (0.5 mg total dissolved solids [tds]) or levodopa (100 mg tds) and had serial ^{123}I-β-CIT SPECT during a 4-year period. Patients treated initially with pramipexole (n = 42) showed a significantly slower mean relative decline of striatal uptake compared with subjects treated initially with levodopa (n = 40) at 2 (47%), 3 (44%), and 4 (37%) years.[31] ELLDOPA is a multicenter, dosage-ranging, controlled clinical trial conducted at 38 sites in the United States and Canada, involving 361 patients with early PD who were randomized to treatment with 150, 300, or 600 mg L-dopa or placebo for 40 weeks. Loss of striatal ^{123}I-β-CIT uptake was significantly greater in the group treated with 600 mg levodopa compared with placebo if subjects with normal imaging were excluded. This study, although limited by its short duration and small sample size, suggested that L-dopa treatment results in greater loss of striatal ^{123}I-β-CIT uptake compared with placebo.[32] The use of dopamine SPECT studies in these trials holds promise for future clinical practice.

DRUG-INDUCED PARKINSONISM/ IATROGENIC PARKINSONISM

DIP is the second most common cause of parkinsonism after PD and accounts for about 4% of all patients with parkinsonism. The common offending drugs include typical antipsychotics or neuroleptics; atypical antipsychotics; gastrointestinal motility drugs such as metoclopramide, domperidone, levosulpiride, clebopride, and itopride; calcium channel blockers such as flunarizine and cinnarizine; and antiepileptic drugs such as lithium.[33] It is usually characterized by bradykinesia and rigidity, which is mostly bilateral and symmetric. Concurrent orofacial and limb dyskinesia and akathisia are helpful in diagnosing DIP due to neuroleptics.[34] As there is overlap between the presentation of PD and DIP, they can be clinically indistinguishable. However, molecular imaging studies may be useful to make this differentiation. In pure DIP, DAT scans show symmetric uptake of radiotracer in bilateral striata. PD can be diagnosed in DIP when the DAT uptake decreases asymmetrically in the striatum.

Lorberboym and colleagues[35] evaluated 20 patients who developed parkinsonism while on neuroleptic agents and 10 age-matched controls. There were 9 patients who had normal scan results and 11 who showed significantly diminished striatal binding, indicating that DIP can be clinically indistinguishable from PD and that SPECT studies help to determine whether these conditions are entirely drug induced or an exacerbation of subclinical. Booij and colleagues[36] noted diminished nigrostriatal dopaminergic cell uptake in PD but not in DIP.

ESSENTIAL TREMOR

ET is defined as an isolated postural/action tremor in otherwise neurologically healthy person. It has been mentioned that up to 25% of patients who were initially diagnosed as having PD were later proved to have ET.[37] ET usually presents as a slowly progressive and kinetic tremor of the upper limbs.[38] It occurs due to abnormalities of central oscillators arising within the olivocerebellar and thalamocortical loops[39] and is not associated with neurodegeneration. Isaias and colleagues[40] proved using [123I]ioflupane that patients with ET had higher uptake values at the putamen and caudate nucleus compared with those with PD but lower than healthy subjects. Benamer and colleagues[41] found that FP-CIT has 95% sensitivity and 93% specificity in differentiating between parkinsonism syndrome and ET.

DEMENTIA WITH LEWY BODIES AND DOPAMINE SPECT

Clinical features for the diagnosis of DLB include fluctuating cognition with pronounced variation of attention and alertness; visual hallucinations that are recurrent, persistent, and well formed; and

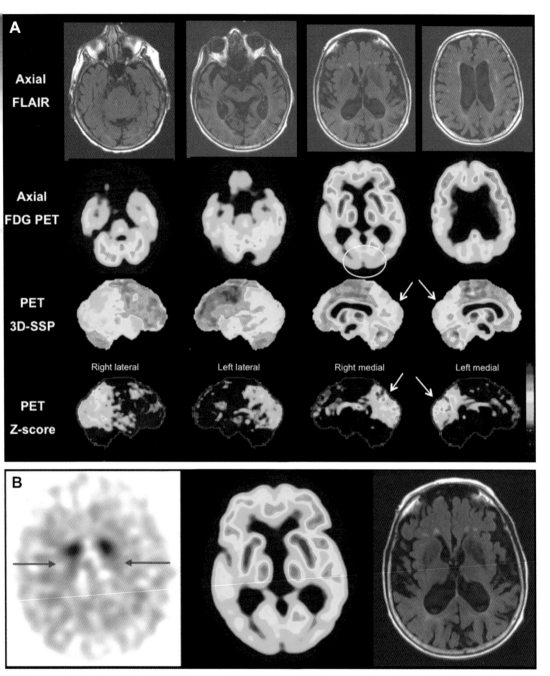

Fig. 5. Lewy body dementia. (*A*) This 76-year-old man presented for evaluation of cognitive dysfunction. In the past 1 to 2 years, the patient's wife noted progressive memory difficulties, forgetfulness, and becoming lost easily when driving. The patient was treated for presumed Alzheimer disease without significant improvement and sought a second opinion. Subspecialty neurology evaluation yielded occasional visual symptoms. MR imaging demonstrates marked diffuse cerebral and cerebellar volume loss. Fludeoxyglucose F 18 (FDG) PET images demonstrate severe temporal, parietal, and occipital hypometabolism. Significant visual cortex hypometabolism is noted (*circle*). Quantitative analysis of FDG PET brain confirms moderately severe visual cortex hypometabolism (*white arrows*). (*B*) DaT scan demonstrates bilaterally absent putamen uptake (*red arrows*) despite preserved metabolism on PET and structural integrity on MR imaging. Final diagnosis is Lewy body dementia. FLAIR, fluid-attenuated inversion recovery; SSP, stereotactic surface projection.

spontaneous (non–drug-induced) parkinsonism.[42] Clinical diagnostic criteria have shown high specificity (>80%) but very low sensitivity (<30%) when compared with autopsy results.[43]

[123I] FP-CIT SPECT is helpful for differentiating DLB and dementia from other causes such as AD (**Fig. 5**). Lewy bodies pathology and concomitant nigrostriatal degeneration are paralleled by a significant loss of presynaptic dopaminergic transporters in the striatum,[44] which can be detected by [123I]FP-CIT SPECT scan. Walker and colleagues[45] studied 20 patients with dementia and noted that the sensitivity of an initial clinical diagnosis of DLB was 75% and specificity was 42%, the sensitivity of the [123I]-2beta-carbometoxy-3beta-(4-iodophenyl)-N-(3-fluoropropyl) nortropane (FP-CIT; ioflupane) scan for the diagnosis of DLB was 88% and specificity was 100%.

A phase III multicenter study was conducted by McKeith and colleagues[46] using [123I]FP-CIT SPECT to confirm the high correlation between abnormal (low-binding) DAT activity and a clinical diagnosis of probable DLB. They assessed 326 patients with clinical diagnoses of probable (n = 94) or possible (n = 57) DLB or non-DLB dementia (n = 147) established by a consensus panel and 3 readers, unaware of the clinical diagnosis, and classified the images as normal or abnormal by visual inspection. Abnormal scan results had a mean sensitivity of 77.7% for detecting clinical probable DLB, with specificity of 90.4% for excluding non-DLB dementia, which was predominantly due to AD. A positive predictive value of 82.4%, negative predictive value of 87.5%, and overall diagnostic accuracy of 85.7% was achieved. Interreader agreement for rating scan results as normal or abnormal was high (Cohen κ = 0.87). Hence, dopamine SPECT is an invaluable tool differentiating DLB from other causes of dementia such as AD.

SUMMARY

The diagnosis of PD and DLB is often not straightforward. When symptoms of PD are atypical or overlap with other diseases (eg, ET or drug induced), [123I]FP-CIT SPECT can improve the diagnostic accuracy. The potential side effects of medications for PD may be avoided, if [123I]FP-CIT SPECT result is normal. [123I]FP-CIT SPECT is helpful in the diagnosis of DLB, differentiating it from other causes of dementia, such as AD.

REFERENCES

1. Gelb DJ, Oliver E, Gilman S. Diagnostic criteria for Parkinson disease. Arch Neurol 1999;56(1):33–9.

2. Tanner CM, Goldman SM. Epidemiology of Parkinson's disease. Neurol Clin 1996;14(2):317–35.

3. Marsden CD. Parkinson's disease. J Neurol Neurosurg Psychiatr 1994;57(6):672–81.

4. Hague SM, Klaffke S, Bandmann O. Neurodegenerative disorders: Parkinson's disease and Huntington's disease. J Neurol Neurosurg Psychiatr 2005; 76(8):1058–63.

5. Neumeyer JL, Wang S, Gao Y, et al. N-omega-fluoroalkyl analogs of (1R)-2 beta-carbomethoxy-3 beta-(4-iodophenyl)-tropane (beta-CIT): radiotracers for positron emission tomography and single photon emission computed tomography imaging of dopamine transporters. J Med Chem 1994;37(11):1558–61.

6. Marvin M, Goldenberg PT. Pharmaceutical Approval Update 2011;36(3):162–4. PMCID: PMC3086106.

7. Ciliax BJ, Heilman C, Demchyshyn LL, et al. The dopamine transporter: immunochemical characterization and localization in brain. J Neurosci 1995; 15(3 Pt 1):1714–23.

8. Kish SJ, Shannak K, Hornykiewicz O. Uneven pattern of dopamine loss in the striatum of patients with idiopathic Parkinson's disease. Pathophysiologic and clinical implications. N Engl J Med 1988; 318(14):876–80.

9. Varrone A, Sansone V, Pellecchia MT, et al. Comparison between a dual-head and a brain-dedicated SPECT system in the measurement of the loss of dopamine transporters with [123I]FP-CIT. Eur J Nucl Med Mol Imaging 2008;35(7):1343–9.

10. Darcourt J, Booij J, Tatsch K, et al. EANM procedure guidelines for brain neurotransmission SPECT using (123)I-labelled dopamine transporter ligands, version 2. Eur J Nucl Med Mol Imaging 2010;37(2):443–50.

11. Booij J, Kemp P. Dopamine transporter imaging with [(123)I]FP-CIT SPECT: potential effects of drugs. Eur J Nucl Med Mol Imaging 2008;35(2):424–38.

12. Morton RJ, Guy MJ, Clauss R, et al. Comparison of different methods of DatSCAN quantification. Nucl Med Commun 2005;26(12):1139–46.

13. Fearnley JM, Lees AJ. Ageing and Parkinson's disease: substantia nigra regional selectivity. Brain 1991;114(Pt 5):2283–301.

14. Marek KL, Seibyl JP, Zoghbi SS, et al. [123I] beta-CIT/SPECT imaging demonstrates bilateral loss of dopamine transporters in hemi-Parkinson's disease. Neurology 1996;46(1):231–7.

15. Vlaar AM, van Kroonenburgh MJ, Kessels AG, et al. Meta-analysis of the literature on diagnostic accuracy of SPECT in parkinsonian syndromes. BMC Neurol 2007;7:27.

16. Asenbaum S, Pirker W, Angelberger P, et al. [123I] beta-CIT and SPECT in essential tremor and Parkinson's disease. J Neural Transm 1998;105(10–12): 1213–28.

17. Haapaniemi TH, Ahonen A, Torniainen P, et al. [123I] beta-CIT SPECT demonstrates decreased brain

dopamine and serotonin transporter levels in untreated parkinsonian patients. Mov Disord 2001; 16(1):124–30.

18. Huang WS, Lin SZ, Lin JC, et al. Evaluation of early-stage Parkinson's disease with 99mTc-TRODAT-1 imaging. J Nucl Med 2001;42(9):1303–8.

19. Muller T, Farahati J, Kuhn W, et al. [123I]beta-CIT SPECT visualizes dopamine transporter loss in de novo parkinsonian patients. Eur Neurol 1998;39(1): 44–8.

20. Schwarz J, Linke R, Kerner M, et al. Striatal dopamine transporter binding assessed by [I-123]IPT and single photon emission computed tomography in patients with early Parkinson's disease: implications for a preclinical diagnosis. Arch Neurol 2000; 57(2):205–8.

21. Van Laere K, De Ceuninck L, Dom R, et al. Dopamine transporter SPECT using fast kinetic ligands: 123I-FP-beta-CIT versus 99mTc-TRODAT-1. Eur J Nucl Med Mol Imaging 2004;31(8):1119–27.

22. Parkinson Study Group. A controlled trial of rasagiline in early Parkinson disease: the TEMPO Study. Arch Neurol 2002;59(12):1937–43.

23. Fahn S, Oakes D, Shoulson I, et al. Levodopa and the progression of Parkinson's disease. N Engl J Med 2004;351(24):2498–508.

24. Morrish PK, Sawle GV, Brooks DJ. An [18F]dopa-PET and clinical study of the rate of progression in Parkinson's disease. Brain 1996;119(Pt 2):585–91.

25. Pirker W, Djamshidian S, Asenbaum S, et al. Progression of dopaminergic degeneration in Parkinson's disease and atypical parkinsonism: a longitudinal beta-CIT SPECT study. Mov Disord 2002;17(1):45–53.

26. Chouker M, Tatsch K, Linke R, et al. Striatal dopamine transporter binding in early to moderately advanced Parkinson's disease: monitoring of disease progression over 2 years. Nucl Med Commun 2001;22(6):721–5.

27. Staffen W, Mair A, Unterrainer J, et al. Measuring the progression of idiopathic Parkinson's disease with [123I] beta-CIT SPECT. J Neural Transm 2000; 107(5):543–52.

28. Innis RB, Marek KL, Sheff K, et al. Effect of treatment with L-dopa/carbidopa or L-selegiline on striatal dopamine transporter SPECT imaging with [123I] beta-CIT. Mov Disord 1999;14(3):436–42.

29. The Parkinson's Progression Markers Initiative (PPMI). 2010. Prog Neurobiol 2011;95(4):629–35. http://dx.doi.org/10.1016/j.pneurobio.2011.09.005. Epub 2011 Sep 14.

30. Jann MW. Advanced strategies for treatment of Parkinson's disease: the role of early treatment. Am J Manag Care 2011;17(Suppl 12):S315–21.

31. Parkinson Study Group. Dopamine transporter brain imaging to assess the effects of pramipexole vs levodopa on Parkinson disease progression. JAMA 2002;287(13):1653–61.

32. Fahn S, Parkinson Study Group. Does levodopa slow or hasten the rate of progression of Parkinson's disease? J Neurol 2005;252(Suppl 4):IV37–42.

33. Shin HW, Chung SJ. Drug-induced parkinsonism. J Clin Neurol 2012;8(1):15–21.

34. Hardie RJ, Lees AJ. Neuroleptic-induced Parkinson's syndrome: clinical features and results of treatment with levodopa. J Neurol Neurosurg Psychiatr 1988;51(6):850–4.

35. Lorberboym M, Treves TA, Melamed E, et al. [123I]-FP/CIT SPECT imaging for distinguishing drug-induced parkinsonism from Parkinson's disease. Mov Disord 2006;21(4):510–4.

36. Booij J, Speelman JD, Horstink MW, et al. The clinical benefit of imaging striatal dopamine transporters with [123I]FP-CIT SPET in differentiating patients with presynaptic parkinsonism from those with other forms of parkinsonism. Eur J Nucl Med 2001;28(3):266–72.

37. Gerasimou G, Costa DC, Papanastasiou E, et al. SPECT study with I-123-ioflupane (DaTSCAN) in patients with essential tremor. Is there any correlation with Parkinson's disease? Ann Nucl Med 2012; 26(4):337–44.

38. Elble RJ, Tremor Research Group. Report from a U.S. conference on essential tremor. Mov Disord 2006;21(12):2052–61.

39. Jenkins IH, Bain PG, Colebatch JG, et al. A positron emission tomography study of essential tremor: evidence for overactivity of cerebellar connections. Ann Neurol 1993;34(1):82–90.

40. Isaias IU, Canesi M, Benti R, et al. Striatal dopamine transporter abnormalities in patients with essential tremor. Nucl Med Commun 2008;29(4):349–53.

41. Benamer TS, Patterson J, Grosset DG, et al. Accurate differentiation of parkinsonism and essential tremor using visual assessment of [123I]-FP-CIT SPECT imaging: the [123I]-FP-CIT study group. Mov Disord 2000;15(3):503–10.

42. McKeith I, Mintzer J, Aarsland D, et al. Dementia with Lewy bodies. Lancet Neurol 2004;3(1):19–28.

43. Lopez OL, Becker JT, Kaufer DI, et al. Research evaluation and prospective diagnosis of dementia with Lewy bodies. Arch Neurol 2002;59(1):43–6.

44. Piggott MA, Marshall EF, Thomas N, et al. Striatal dopaminergic markers in dementia with Lewy bodies, Alzheimer's and Parkinson's diseases: rostrocaudal distribution. Brain 1999;122(Pt 8):1449–68.

45. Walker Z, Jaros E, Walker RW, et al. Dementia with Lewy bodies: a comparison of clinical diagnosis, FP-CIT single photon emission computed tomography imaging and autopsy. J Neurol Neurosurg Psychiatr 2007;78(11):1176–81.

46. McKeith I, O'Brien J, Walker Z, et al. Sensitivity and specificity of dopamine transporter imaging with 123I-FP-CIT SPECT in dementia with Lewy bodies: a phase III, multicentre study. Lancet Neurol 2007; 6(4):305–13.

Dopamine
PET Imaging and Parkinson Disease

Shichun Peng, PhD[a], Doris J. Doudet, PhD[b],
Vijay Dhawan, PhD[a], Yilong Ma, PhD[a],*

KEYWORDS

- Neurodegenerative disorders • Parkinsonism • Dopamine • PET • Imaging biomarkers • Diagnosis
- Disease progression • Therapeutic intervention

KEY POINTS

- Dopamine (DA)-specific PET radioligands provide viable imaging biomarkers to describe dysfunctional molecular substrates underlying Parkinson disease (PD) and parkinsonian disorders.
- Presynaptic DA markers allow accurate discrimination of idiopathic PD from atypical PD and correlate with the severity of clinical symptoms in individual patients.
- Postsynaptic DA markers enable quantitative measurement of endogenous DA release in challenging conditions.
- Longitudinal changes in these DA markers have revealed critical insights on the neurobiological mechanisms associated with compensatory processes in the brain and therapeutic efficacy in clinical trials.

INTRODUCTION

Parkinson disease (PD) is a major movement disorder resulting from the progressive degeneration of dopaminergic (DA) neurons in the nigrostriatal system, as well as non-DA neurons of serotonergic and noradrenergic origins in the brainstem and their related neural pathways. The loss of nigral neurons leads to the deficiency of dopamine (DA), a monoamine neurotransmitter, and is the basis of DA replacement therapy with medications or cellular regenerative interventions. The loss of serotoninergic and noradrenergic innervations may play a role in several nonmotor symptoms such as mood and sleep disorders. Although these neuronal deficits are often confined in a few isolated neurochemical pathways, they have significant consequences on the integrity of the brain by way of the widespread interconnectivity among various brain circuits. It is this systemic impairment in functional and anatomic substrates that underlies motor and nonmotor symptoms in PD.[1,2] Despite progressive striatal depletion, there is an extended presymptomatic phase in individual patients, implying a sustained compensation process in the brain. Recent research suggests that onset of motor symptoms may be associated with the failure of such preclinical compensatory mechanisms in PD.[3]

The diagnosis of idiopathic PD is based chiefly on the clinical manifestations of motor symptoms of resting tremor, rigidity, bradykinesia, and postural instability. The diagnostic decision is often complicated by the similarity of symptoms in early patients with atypical parkinsonian disorders such as multiple system atrophy (MSA), progressive

Disclosure: The authors have nothing to disclose.

Support: This work was supported in part by NIH R01 NS 35069, R01 NS 32368, P50 NS 38370 and the General Clinical Research Center (M01 RR 018535) and the Morris K. Udall Center of Excellence for PD Research (P50 NS 71675) at The Feinstein Institute for Medical Research.

[a] Center for Neurosciences, The Feinstein Institute for Medical Research, 350 Community Drive, Manhasset, NY 11030, USA; [b] Department of Neurology, University of British Columbia, 2221 Wesbrook Mall, Vancouver, British Columbia V2Z 2J9, Canada
* Corresponding author.
E-mail address: yma@nshs.edu

PET Clin 8 (2013) 469–485
http://dx.doi.org/10.1016/j.cpet.2013.08.003
1556-8598/13/$ – see front matter © 2013 Elsevier Inc. All rights reserved.

supranuclear palsy (PSP), and corticobasal ganglionic degeneration (CBGD). A misdiagnosis can significantly affect clinical management of patients over the early course of the disease. A definitive clinical diagnosis can only be established in patients by long-term follow-up of 2 to 4 years by experienced movement disorder specialists. Although quantitative rating scales have been used to quantify the severity of clinical symptoms in patients, they are subjective and unable to detect any covert changes during preclinical stages, and they are often insensitive to early signs of disease onset. It is therefore difficult to accurately distinguish idiopathic PD from atypical PD on clinical grounds alone.

A wide variety of novel radiotracers have been developed to characterize DA and non-DA dysfunction in PD using both positron emission tomography (PET) and single-photon emission computed tomography (SPECT). Specific neurochemical indicators of the disease process may be measured more directly using radioligands that target particular neurotransmitters, neurotransporters, and neuroreceptors. By contrast, complementary information on the disease-mediated functional changes may be extracted indirectly in terms of regional differences in cerebral perfusion and metabolism over the brain. In particular, this effort is directed toward the identification and validation of disease-specific descriptors that can serve as imaging biomarkers for clinical and biomedical translational studies. A viable imaging biomarker should ideally meet the conditions summarized in **Box 1**.

The applications of non–DA-specific imaging methods in PD have previously been reviewed

from the perspectives of neurochemistry[4] and cerebral blood flow and metabolism.[5] It has been reported that brain network analysis of 2-deoxy-2-[^{18}F]fluoro-D-glucose (FDG) PET images can provide characteristic metabolic patterns to distinguish patients with idiopathic PD or atypical PD from healthy volunteers. Monkeys with specific 1-methyl-4-phenyl-1,2,3,6-tetrahydropyridine (MPTP)–induced DA nigral lesions display the same metabolic pattern as patients with PD.[6] The expression of these disease-specific brain networks can be measured prospectively on a single-case basis in individual subjects. Many studies with FDG-PET imaging have been published in recent years and suggest that network scores seem to fulfill the key criteria to serve as viable imaging biomarkers (see Ref.[7]).

This article describes the latest development in major DA-related radioligands and imaging techniques that are used clinically in human subjects and parkinsonian patients. The emphasis of the article is on the resting-state studies in PD populations without dementia. The article begins with a brief introduction to the normal neuroanatomy involved in DA projection systems. It also summarizes practical imaging protocols and the optimal analytical methods designed to simplify the implementation of these imaging techniques for clinical and research applications. The article focuses on their use in providing imaging biomarkers for diagnosis, progression, and treatment response.

NORMAL ANATOMY/IMAGING TECHNIQUE

There are 4 major pathways involved in the neurotransmission of DA in the brain: the mesolimbic, mesocortical, nigrostriatal, and tuberoinfundibular pathways. Each of these pathways has a distinctive connection with the subdivisions of the striatum. The putamen is mainly involved in motor function, whereas the ventral striatum and the caudate nucleus are primarily involved in limbic and cognitive processes. In addition, there is a gradient of DA motor innervation in the striatal subregions. This gradient is evident in the degeneration of the nigral neurons in the substantia nigra pars compacta in PD leading to a loss of DA terminals, beginning in the posterior putamen and, as the disease progresses, spreading gradually to the anterior putamen and caudate nucleus, but mostly sparing the ventral striatum. Imaging of DA radiotracers reveals vital information on the integrity of the nigrostriatal projection systems and related cortical pathways from the perspective of presynaptic and postsynaptic DA function. DA-specific radioligands are designed to have fast, high, and selective accumulation in the target

---

Box 1
Criteria for a viable imaging biomarker for neurodegenerative disorders

- High sensitivity and specificity for detecting disease onset and for early differential diagnosis

- Clinical correlation with independent measures of disease severity or behavioral abnormality

- High sensitivity to track longitudinal change over the time course of disease progression

- High accuracy to assess therapeutic responses and correlations with clinical outcome measures

- High test-retest reliability in patients within an imaging center and excellent reproducibility in independent patients across different imaging centers

brain region with rapid washout in the nonspecific reference region. Many optimal imaging protocols and analytical methods have also been devised for accurately measuring parameters of neurobiological interest in the brain.

Presynaptic Dopaminergic Function

Dopamine synthesis
Assay of 6-[18F]fluoro-L-dopa (FDOPA) can provide a sensitive measure of synthesis, storage, and turnover of DA in presynaptic DA nerve terminals.[8–12] FDOPA PET imaging reflects the activity of aromatic amino acid decarboxylase (AADC), an enzyme largely responsible for catalyzing the conversion of L-dopa into DA.[13,14] Other radiofluorinated L-m-tyrosines, including 6-[18F]fluoro-L-m-tyrosine ([18F]FMT), are also substrates of AADC and provide an index of DA synthesis and storage,[15,16] but do not undergo the same metabolic fate and do not provide information on DA turnover.[17]

Dopamine transporter
Dopamine transporter (DAT) is responsible for the regulation of synaptic reuptake of DA in the nigrostriatal projection systems. Cocaine analogues based on tropanes like [11C]-labeled 2β-carbomethoxy-3β-(4-fluorophenyl)tropane ([11C]CFT) or methylphenidate ([11C]MP) and [18F]-labeled N-3-fluoropropyl-2-β-carboxymethoxy-3-β-(4-iodophenyl)nortropane ([18F]FPCIT) are among the radioligands most commonly used for PET imaging of presynaptic DA nerve terminals in humans.[18–20] Imaging of DAT has become more widely available with the use of commercial SPECT radioligands, also from the tropane family, such as [123I]-labeled (1R)-2-β-carbomethoxy-3-β-(4-iodophenyl)-tropane ([123I]β-CIT)[21] and its fluoroalkyl esters [123I] FPCIT.[22] DAT binding seems to be unaffected by L-dopa treatment in monkey studies with SPECT and postmortem examination.[23]

Vesicular monoamine transporter type 2
Vesicular monoamine transporter type 2 (VMAT2) is the transporter responsible for packing monoamine neurotransmitters (DA, serotonin, and noradrenaline) from the cytoplasm into vesicles for storage and subsequent synaptic release. [11C]dihydrotetrabenazine (DTBZ) can be used as a reliable measure of monoaminergic nerve terminal density.[24] More recently, [18F]-labeled 9-fluoropropyl-(1)-DTBZ ([18F]AV-133) has been successfully synthesized as a higher affinity fluoropropyl derivative of DTBZ.[25] VMAT2 binding seems to be less sensitive to drug-mediated or lesion-mediated regulation than other presynaptic ligands[26] but it is not completely insensitive.[27]

However, this method has a lower signal/noise ratio than FDOPA uptake and DAT binding, but does not have specificity for DA terminals.[2]

Postsynaptic Dopaminergic Function
Radioligands such as [11C]raclopride and [11C] N-methylspiperone can provide sensitive measures of local DA D2 receptor density in the striatum. Newer tracers such as [11C]-labeled (S)-N-((1-Ethyl-2-pyrrolidinyl)methyl)-5-bromo-2-[11C]methoxy-3-methoxybenzamide ([11C]FLB 457) and [18F]fallypride are more sensitive in detecting changes in D2 receptor binding in extrastriatal regions such as prefrontal and anterior cingulate cortices during the performance of cognitive functional tasks in normal subjects.[28,29] Because ligands of the benzamide family have limited affinity for the D2 receptors and compete with the endogenous ligand for the binding sites, changes in their binding potential reflect variations in endogenous DA levels in challenge situations. PET studies of these tracers have shown striatal and prefrontal DA release in response to behavioral activations[30,31] and pharmacologic stimulations[32,33] in healthy volunteers.

In developing and validating the neurobiological usefulness of a novel DA-specific radioligand it is often necessary to define its brain distribution in subcortical and cortical structures in healthy volunteers. An age-related decline of 5% to 8% per decade is observed in striatal regions of normal controls and monkeys in most of the markers of DA function described earlier.[24,34,35] Age-related changes in FDOPA uptake are absent as a result of AADC upregulation in the aged DA terminals. The normative database can provide the magnitude and range in regional uptake/binding of the radioligand as a function of healthy aging. This information is necessary for accurately detecting functional abnormality on a single-case basis in individual patients. **Table 1** gives a summary of the most commonly used radiotracers and references cited throughout the text.

Imaging Protocols and Analytical Methods
The salient features of imaging protocols for DA-related PET radioligands are included in **Box 2**. PET images are typically acquired in dynamic mode up to a period of 60/120 minutes for [11C]-labeled or [18F]-labeled radioligands immediately after intravenous radiotracer injection. Imaging with [11C]-based radioligands usually affords a higher injected dose and shorter scanning duration to compensate for the rapid decay of radioactivity caused by their shorter half-lives. In contrast, imaging with [18F]-based radioligands generally

Table 1
PET radioligands for imaging dopaminergic function in PD

Radiolabel	Radiotracers	References
AADC		
F18	FDOPA	8–14,17,22,35–37, 43,44,48,49,52, 56–60,63–65, 70,73–75,77, 78,81,85
F18	FMT	15–17,83,84
DAT		
C11	CFT	18,40,65,86
C11	MP	19,34–37,41,56, 70,74,77,88
C11	FECIT	46
C11	PE2I	57
F18	FPCIT	20,50,62,71,72
VMAT2		
C11	DTBZ	24,26,35–37,41, 56,64,65,70, 74,76,77,88
F18	AV-133	25,45,47
D2 receptor		
C11	Raclopride	11,30–32,34,41, 57,66–68,76, 79,85–87
C11	FLB 457	28,69
F18	Fallypride	29,33
F18	Desmethoxyfally-pride	51

Abbreviations: FECIT, 2-β-carbomethoxy-3-β-(4-fluorophenyl)-tropane; PE2I, N-(3-iodoprop-2 E-enyl)-2β-carbomethoxy-3β-(4-methylphenyl)nortropane.

Box 2
Imaging protocols for DA-specific PET radioligands

- The participants are scanned following at least 12 hours off medications of L-dopa and other central nervous system (CNS) drugs
- Radiotracers (5–15 mCi/185–555 MBq) are administrated intravenously either as a single bolus or by continuous infusion over a period of time
- Dynamic imaging usually starts immediately after radiotracer administration and consists of a set of contiguous frames beginning with finer sampling over early times and ending with longer sampling over late times
- As an alternative, static image(s) may be acquired over a predetermined time window when the radiotracer reaches a steady-state equilibrium in uptake/binding
- Photon attenuation correction data are obtained using transmission images acquired either before or after the administration of radiotracers, which is performed with PET with point sources or with the computed tomography (CT) part of a PET/CT depending on the configuration of imaging systems

time. Attenuation is usually corrected using an attenuation map measured from a transmission scan acquired either before or after the administration of the radiotracer for a dedicated PET camera. For a PET/computed tomography (CT) scanner, this is achieved with a low-energy CT scan, adjusted for energy differences relative to positron-emitting radiopharmaceutical agents. The projection data are then reconstructed into three-dimensional image volumes with analytical methods based on filtered back projection or iterative methods based on ordered subsets expectation maximization algorithms.

In addition to the clinical use for visualizing functional abnormality, PET images are mostly analyzed to extract neurobiological parameters representing uptake or binding of radioligands in the brain. Over the last 2 decades, analytical techniques have evolved from absolute quantification with input functions derived from arterial blood sampling or dynamic imaging procedures to semiquantitative measures with the use of reference tissue models.[38–42] Brain regions chosen as a reference tissue tend to be occipital lobe or cerebellum, known to have low to negligible binding sites for specific DA radioligands, which is best confirmed by postmortem analysis of particular imaging agents such as VMAT2

requires a lower injected dose to compensate for higher dosimetry, longer scanning duration, but higher signal/noise ratio because of their longer half-lives. [^{18}F]-based radioligands offer the unique ability for easy distribution of radiotracers from a cyclotron facility to satellite sites nearby. However, from a research perspective, with [^{11}C]-labeled ligands, more than one radiotracer may be administered to a single subject in a day, leading to combined rapid evaluation of multiple aspects of the DA system.[36,37]

The time sampling is shorter early but is gradually increased at late times in accordance with the unique uptake characteristics of each particular radiotracer. Projection data from dynamic acquisition are corrected online for physical effects of photo attenuation, scatter, randoms, detector efficiency variation, and electronic dead

protein in human brains.[27] Both multiple-time graphical analyses and target/background ratio methods are simple, but valuable in estimating parameters of interest for disease discrimination and clinical correlation.[43–45]

Two general approaches have been in use by clinicians and biomedical investigators. The first method is based on the analysis of images over a set of predefined volumes of interest (VOIs). This hypothesis-driven approach is most suitable for quantifying regional neurobiological parameters in the native space of each brain. The second method is based on the brain mapping analysis of images in a standard anatomic space to provide complementary information on disease-mediated changes in these measures over the brain. This data-driven approach is most useful for localizing brain regions showing functional abnormality or clinical correlates without an a priori hypothesis.

In recent years, it has become feasible to simplify imaging protocols from dynamic to static acquisition at later stages following radiotracer administration. A simple method of standardized uptake value ratio can be used for image analysis when the uptake of a tracer establishes a steady state.[43–45] As a result, imaging acquisition for this type of radioligands can be conducted like an FDG-PET study. Scanning can begin after the subjects complete the necessary period of radiotracer uptake off the scanner. This simplification increases compliance, especially in patients with severe disability, decreases the patient discomfort associated with a longer scanning session, and increases the throughput in the imaging facility.

IMAGING FINDINGS/PATHOLOGY

Clinicians identify patients with idiopathic PD by the appearance of at least 2 of the 4 cardinal motor features described earlier. The patients are evaluated clinically in the practically defined Off state with Unified Parkinson Disease Rating Scale (UPDRS), Hoehn and Yahr Scale (HY), and Schwab and England Activities of Daily Living (ADL) Scale. In general, a higher score on one or more of these scales is associated with a longer disease duration in an individual patient. Such ratings are less useful in patients showing the earliest signs of motor dysfunction but more useful in patients confirmed to have idiopathic PD. In particular, these measures may not be sensitive enough to reflect subtle incremental changes resulting from disease progression and following neuroprotective or symptomatic therapies. Early patients with atypical parkinsonism similarly may not be separated adequately by clinical rating scales.

The molecular imaging modality with DA-specific PET radioligands has played important roles in the assessment of PD pathophysiology and differential diagnosis between idiopathic and atypical patients with PD, and for the evaluation of the efficacy of novel experimental therapeutics. Among presynaptic DA markers, FDOPA uptake and DAT binding are used more frequently, followed by VMAT2 binding. In contrast, D2 receptor binding is the most common postsynaptic DA marker. This marker alone is not particularly useful for diagnosis purposes, but is valuable in combination with FDOPA/DAT or for measuring endogenous DA release. Both VOI-based and voxel-based analytical methods are often used either separately or concurrently in practice.[31,46,47] Basic information for physicians considering the use of DA-specific imaging is presented in **Box 3**.

Disease Diagnosis

In addition to the onset of motor symptoms and a good response to L-dopa ($\geq$20% improvement in UPDRS motor ratings), nonmedicated, early patients with hemi-idiopathic PD (HY 1–1.5) may be identified by an anteroposterior gradient of tracer uptake, and asymmetric uptake on PET scans. A 50% to 60 % reduction in FDOPA uptake (**Fig. 1**)

Box 3
What the referring physician needs to know

- At the time of imaging, the patients have had to withdraw from L-dopa or DA agonists for at least 12 hours and are not taking other CNS medications, such as neuroleptics

- There may be large intraindividual and interindividual variability in DA-specific imaging outcomes because of differences in subject age and possibly gender

- DA-specific imaging markers decrease with subject age, and comparison with age-matched database values is necessary for adequate interpretation

- Severity of clinical symptoms may be associated with lower image quality in elderly subjects or patients with advanced disease

- Differential diagnosis of idiopathic or atypical PD may be confirmed clinically over a follow-up period of at least 2 years or/and by the striatal distribution pattern of the presynaptic DA tracer

- Some individuals with normal presynaptic nigrostriatal DA function may show signs of manifesting parkinsonism, such as essential tremor and dystonic tremor, over the early course of the disease

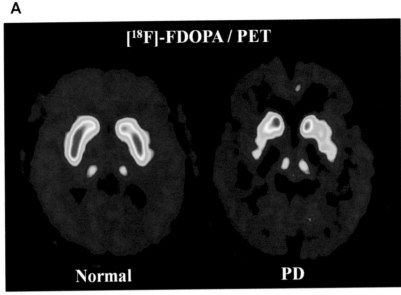

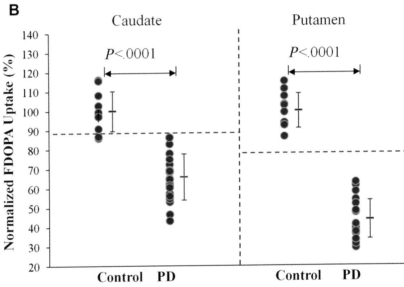

Fig. 1. (*A*) FDOPA PET images in healthy volunteers and patients with idiopathic PD. (*B*) FDOPA uptake is reduced in caudate and putamen to discriminate the patients from the healthy volunteers. (*Data from* Dhawan V, Ma Y, Pillai V, et al. Comparative analysis of striatal FDOPA uptake in Parkinson's disease: ratio method versus graphical approach. J Nucl Med 2002;43:1327; with permission.)

is commonly found in the posterior putamen (symptomatic hemisphere) contralateral to the clinically affected body side.[44] Extrastriatal reductions in FDOPA uptake are seen in cortical motor areas, even in early disease.[48] Frontal association areas are also affected in later disease but limbic areas are less affected. Many studies with a variety of DAT ligands report similar patterns of bilateral, asymmetrical reduction in striatal DAT binding in patients with PD at early stages (**Fig. 2**A) with both PET[18,20,36,46] and SPECT.[21]

DA radioligands have also been used to measure disease-related decline in nigrostriatal VMAT2 binding (**Fig. 3**A). Specific DTBZ binding is variably reduced in various striatal and brainstem regions in patients with PD.[24] Striatal and midbrain DTBZ binding is asymmetric in patients with early PD, with greatest reductions (up to 73%) contralateral to the most clinically affected limbs indicating a substantial preclinical nigrostriatal disorder. The main characteristics of abnormal VMAT2 binding in patients revealed by DTBZ have been replicated

A

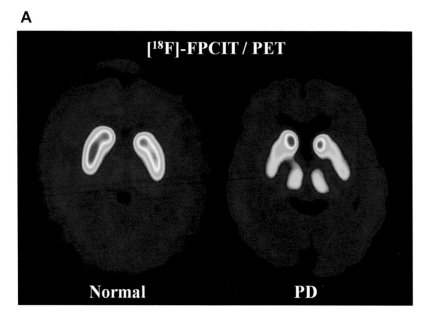

B

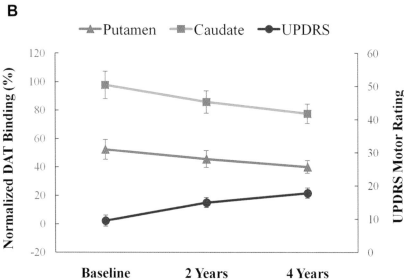

Fig. 2. (*A*) FPCIT PET images in healthy volunteers and patients with idiopathic PD. DAT binding is reduced in caudate and putamen to discriminate the patients from the healthy volunteers. (*B*) Increased motor symptoms and progressive reduction in presynaptic DA biomarker in patients with idiopathic PD measured with FPCIT PET. (*Data from* Huang C, Tang C, Feigin A, et al. Changes in network activity with the progression of Parkinson's disease. Brain 2007;130:1838–9; with permission.)

more recently with [^{18}F]AV-133[45,47] as well as in postmortem analysis.[27] The diagnostic criteria for PET imaging in PD are given in **Box 4**. Different presynaptic markers show an excellent diagnostic accuracy between early-stage idiopathic PD and healthy controls, with a sensitivity of 95% to 100% and specificity of 90% to 95%.

PET imaging with presynaptic markers has been replicated in nonhuman primate models.[14] One study analyzed FDOPA, MP, and DTBZ images in the same monkeys with mild to severe systemic MPTP lesions.[35] The mean reduction of the binding of the three ligands was variable in the caudate and putamen and depended on the symptom severity. Binding of all three ligands was also variably reduced in the anterior cingulate cortex, brainstem, and thalamus, reflecting toxicity of MPTP for extrastriatal catecholamine innervations.

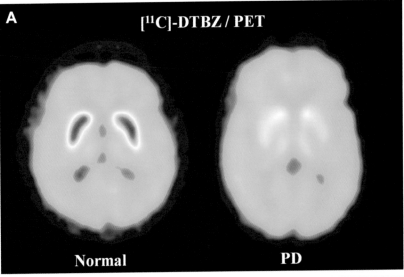

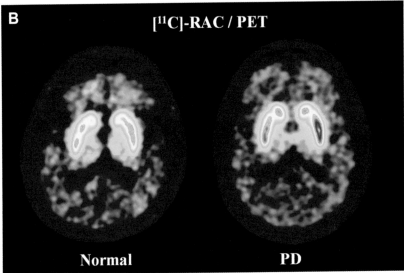

Fig. 3. (*A*) DTBZ PET images in healthy volunteers and patients with idiopathic PD. VMAT2 binding is reduced in caudate and putamen to discriminate the patients from the healthy volunteers. (*B*) Raclopride (RAC) PET images in healthy volunteers and patients with idiopathic PD. Dopamine D2 receptor binding is increased in the putamen of patients with early, unmedicated PD relative to the healthy volunteers. (*Courtesy of* The Pacific Parkinson Research Center, Vancouver, British Columbia, Canada; with permission.)

The differential diagnosis of parkinsonian disorders can be challenging, especially early in the course of the disease. A more accurate distinction between idiopathic and atypical PD would be helpful to inform clinical management of patients and to reduce the number of patients without idiopathic PD enrolled in clinical trials. This is generally facilitated by detecting multigroup differences in striatal uptake/binding values or the ratios between substriatal regions. In patients with idiopathic PD, FDOPA uptake is reduced in the posterior putamen but relatively preserved in the caudate and anterior putamen.[22] By contrast, in patients with atypical

PD, comparable reductions in FDOPA uptake can be observed in both the caudate and putamen.[49] FDOPA PET showed more widespread basal ganglia dysfunction in MSA than in PD with similar disease duration, and extrastriatal loss of DA innervation could be detected in the red nucleus and locus coeruleus. A recent study has shown that variation in DAT binding in striatal subdivisions can be exploited for distinguishing patients with idiopathic and atypical PD with high sensitivity but lower specificity.[50]

Although the measurement of DA D2 receptor density alone is not particularly useful for PD

Box 4
Diagnostic criteria of idiopathic PD

Clinical criteria

PD may be diagnosed clinically by identifying the earliest signs of motor dysfunction and a good response to an acute dose of L-dopa ($\geq$20% improvement in objective disease measures of motor symptoms).

Motor symptoms usually appear unilaterally at disease onset and include resting tremor, rigidity, bradykinesia, and postural instability.

Imaging criteria

PD may be diagnosed with PET imaging by the nonuniform distribution of presynaptic DA markers.

The early-stage PD is characterized by an asymmetry and gradient in presynaptic DA function with the largest reduction in the contralateral dorsal-posterior putamen compared with the caudate nucleus and the ventral-anterior putamen.

A quantitative diagnostic confirmation may be made when striatal DA loss exceeds a certain threshold. The threshold is determined in posterior putamen in reference to a normative database.

Box 5
Differential diagnosis of idiopathic and atypical PD

The differential diagnosis between idiopathic and atypical PD is important for adequate clinical care of patients in early phases of the disease course and for phenotypical patient screening before enrollment in clinical trials.

Key diagnostic features

Presynaptic DA markers may be useful in early detection of idiopathic PD by taking into account the asymmetry of clinical symptoms and the uneven distribution of striatal DA hypofunction.

Patients with atypical PD tend to show symmetric clinical symptoms of parkinsonism with comparable reductions in presynaptic markers in both the caudate and putamen. Patients with MSA develop autonomic symptoms such as severe orthostatic hypotension and cerebellar symptoms like ataxia. By contrast, patients with PSP develop parkinsonism with early postural instability, falls, and oculomotor abnormalities.

Enhancement of diagnostic accuracy

The diagnostic performance can be improved with the use of rigorous statistical metrics such as receiver operating characteristic analysis. The accuracy of differential diagnosis may be enhanced by including other information like intrastrial ratios of imaging markers as additional outcome measures.

---

diagnosis, DA D2 receptor binding allows for the differentiation of patients with idiopathic and atypical PD with high accuracy.[51] This study confirms the relative sparing of D2 receptors in the DA-denervated putamen of idiopathic patients, in contrast with a more substantial loss of striatal DA receptors in atypical patients. However, this differential DA topography is often insufficient to discriminate idiopathic PD from atypical PD at early clinical stages. Furthermore, some (10%–15%) patients have parkinsonian-type motor symptoms but normal DA substrates based on FDOPA PET and DAT SPECT scans,[52,53] a phenomenon nicknamed scans without evidence of DA deficiency [SWEDD] and thought to be related to dystonic tremor.[54] The factors influencing the differential diagnosis are provided in **Box 5**. Although DA imaging with multitracers can improve the accuracy of differential diagnosis,[55] this is usually not cost-effective or feasible outside of research-oriented specialty centers.

PET imaging has revealed both similarities and differences between idiopathic PD and familial PD. An early study found that carriers of PD-specific mutations such as leucine-rich repeat kinase 2 (LRRK2) are nearly indistinguishable

from idiopathic cases on PET markers of DA dysfunction.[56] Both presynaptic and postsynaptic striatal DA markers are reduced to similar levels in patients with early-onset PD with or without mutations of the parkin gene,[57] with FDOPA uptake reduced by 32% and 60% in caudate and putamen, and DAT binding decreased by 44% and 59% compared with normal control values. Further analysis revealed extrastriatal decreases of FDOPA uptake or DAT binding in substantia nigra. The reduction in presynaptic markers was also observed in mutation carriers of PTEN-induced putative kinase 1 (PINK1) causing recessively inherited early-onset PD.[58] Striatal FDOPA uptake declined not only in homozygous mutation carriers but also, to a lesser extent, in the putamen of heterozygous mutation carriers.

Clinical Correlation

A robust imaging biomarker has to show clinical correlations with objective measures of disease severity and cognitive impairment in PD. UPDRS motor ratings correlated consistently with striatal values in presynaptic DA markers such as FDOPA uptake,[43,59] DAT binding,[19,20] and VMAT2 binding.[47] By contrast, striatal reductions in VMAT2 binding correlated significantly with PD duration and SE scores, but not with HY stage or with motor UPDRS subscale scores.[24] The side and severity of DAT/VMAT2 binding reduction significantly correlated with the severity and asymmetry of clinical motor scores.[24,46] In addition, extrastriatal DAT dysfunction could predict the conversion from HY 1 to HY 2.[18]

PET imaging with DA radioligands has also been useful in identifying nonmotor functional abnormality such as cognitive correlates in caudate and putamen. Mental and motor components of executive dysfunction were reported to correlate with FDOPA uptake in the caudate and putamen in patients with advanced PD.[60] DAT binding losses in the putamen correlated with motor and cognitive dysfunction involved in the recognition of emotional gestures in PD.[19] This loss was positively related to the reduction of ventrolateral prefrontal activation. DAT dysfunction in the caudate but not the putamen was associated with resting brain metabolic changes underlying cognitive impairment.[61,62] These studies support the notion that a loss of DA neurotransmission in the putamen/caudate results in impairment in motor and cognition domains.

Several studies have investigated behavioral correlations between PET imaging of presynaptic DA markers and postmortem measurements in MPTP-lesioned nonhuman primate models of experimental parkinsonism. The degree of motor dysfunction correlated negatively with FDOPA uptake and DTBZ binding potential, tyrosine hydroxylase (TH)–immunoreactive cell counts in substantia nigra, striatal DA markers (TH, DAT, and VMAT2), and striatal DA concentration.[14,63,64] There was a critical threshold of nigral cell loss and DA innervation distinguishing between the asymptomatic and symptomatic parkinsonian monkeys. This intoxication protocol established a close correlation between cell loss in the substantia nigra, striatal DA depletion, and the severity of motor symptoms. In monkeys with hemiparkinsonism imaged with FDOPA and tracers of DAT and VMAT2,[65] striatal uptake for each radiotracer correlated strongly with stereological nigral cell counts for nigral loss less than 50% but very strongly with striatal DA over the full range of depletion. This finding may explain differences between neuroimaging and clinical end points reported in some human trials.

Imaging of Endogenous DA

Some D2-specific radiotracers (eg, raclopride) are easily displaced by endogenous DA in challenge conditions, making them suitable for imaging DA release in intact or unaffected DA terminals. For instance, this ability allowed demonstration of reduced DA release in patients with PD in various behavioral and pharmacologic challenges,[32,66] and observation of a placebo effect in patients with PD.[67] DA release in patients with early-stage PD was reduced in the dorsal caudate but preserved in the medial prefrontal cortex during the performance of cognitive tasks related to executive dysfunction.[31] This work shows that executive deficits in patients with early PD are associated with impaired nigrostriatal DA function, resulting in impairment in the corticobasal ganglia circuit, but mesocortical DA transmission seems well preserved in these patients. DA release was also detected in the ventral striatum and in the midbrain in patients with PD with impulse control disorder as a result of treatment with DA agonists,[68,69] showing the abnormal DA processing underlying the medication-induced impulse control disorder in PD.

Disease Progression

Natural history studies of disease progression are critical for assessing the efficacy of neuroprotective and therapeutic trials to prevent continued deterioration in the functional integrity of DA nerve terminals. The former are designed to delay the symptom onset in at-risk populations, whereas the latter are designed to slow the rate of progression in patients. Over the last 10 years, multitracer PET imaging has increasingly been used to follow the degeneration of DA innervation in PD and animal models. This approach has not only offered greater insights on the neurobiological mechanism of neurodegeneration but has also allowed the assessment of the relative performance of PET ligands as potential biomarkers of PD. The pros and cons of DA-specific imaging are listed in **Box 6**.

Many longitudinal studies have been published on neurochemical progression in presynaptic DA integrity in subjects at risk of developing PD and in patients with this disorder. PET studies with FDOPA and tracers of DAT and VMAT2 show that striatal indices in 3 presynaptic DA markers were variably decreased in patients with PD[36] and over the course of progression in asymptomatic members of parkinsonian LKKR2 kindred.[70] Reduced DAT binding was the earliest indication of subclinical DA dysfunction and progression to clinical disease was generally associated with the emergence of abnormal FDOPA uptake.

Box 6
Pearls, pitfalls, and variants

Pearls for DA PET imaging

A single scan acquired some time after radiotracer injection may be sufficient for separating patients with idiopathic PD from healthy controls and patients with atypical PD in a clinical research environment.

Presynaptic DA markers are reduced relative to healthy controls and decreased with the increased severity of clinical symptoms in patients with advanced disease. There is significant correlation between asymmetry of striatal values and clinical asymmetry measured with the motor UPDRS in patients with idiopathic PD.

Atypical patients with PD have more uniform reductions in striatal DA markers compared with healthy controls.

Pitfalls for DA PET imaging

A. Binding to non-DA nerve terminals

FDOPA and VMAT2 are nonspecific to DA and may label noradrenaline. DAT is more specific for DA even though some radiotracers may have very low binding to serotonin transporters.

B. Upregulation: FDOPA, D2 receptor; downregulation: DAT, VMAT2

Most VMAT2 ligands are localized on DA nerve terminals and are less susceptible to compensatory changes during the course of the disease.

C. Influence of medications

DAT and VMAT2 are less affected by antiparkinsonian dopaminergic medications such as L-dopa.

D. Variability of methodological factors

DA-specific markers are influenced by differences in imaging protocols and characteristics of tomographic systems.

Variants for DA PET imaging

Clinical diagnosis and rating scales of the disease may be subjective and depend on medications and the effect of placebo.

Most presynaptic and postsynaptic DA markers decrease with age, leading to lower image quality in older subjects.

Presynaptic DA markers show a flooring effect with disease progression resulting in lower statistical power. DAT is sensitive to the floor effect early on.

Be aware of parkinsonian patients with other forms of secondary parkinsonism or having SWEDD.

In one study, 15 patients initially with hemi-PD with disease duration less than or equal to 2 years were scanned with a DAT tracer and FDG-PET to evaluate longitudinal changes in striatal DAT density and PD-related metabolic brain network (PDRP) expression at baseline and at 2 and 4 years.[71] Increased rates in UPDRS motor ratings correlated with loss rates of striatal DAT binding measured in both caudate and putamen over the course of the follow-up (see **Fig. 2**B). The deterioration of motor symptoms correlated similarly with changes in striatal DAT binding and PDRP network activity. This finding had been replicated when conducting the same analysis separately in hemispheres ipsilateral or contralateral to the more affected limbs based on clinical diagnosis at baseline.[72] Putamen DAT binding in the clinical hemisphere was lower but progressed more slowly compared with the preclinical hemisphere. By contrast, decreased caudate DAT binding or increased PDRP activity was also evident in preclinical hemispheres with rates of change similar to those measured concurrently in clinical hemispheres. Although most work used a linear regression to describe the trajectory of progression over a short interval, a nonlinear decline in FDOPA uptake has been reported in the contralateral putamen, being faster at the beginning of the disease.[73]

In another study, 78 patients and 35 controls were scanned using PET with FDOPA and tracers of DAT and VMAT2 at baseline and 4 and 8 years of follow-up.[74] Greater reductions in the three presynaptic DA markers were related exponentially to longer symptom duration in individual patients. Further, the degree of denervation at disease onset was different between striatal subregions but the relative rate of disease progression was similar among these subregions. Although the anteroposterior gradient of severity was unchanged for DA synthesis, storage, and reuptake, the asymmetry between the more and less affected striatum became less prominent over the disease course. These findings agree with those from DAT binding[71,72] and FDOPA uptake.[59,75]

In a multitracer longitudinal study in MPTP monkeys, an early (2 months) decrease (46%) of striatal VMAT2 in asymptomatic animals preceded changes in DAT and D2 receptors, despite the progressive loss of all presynaptic DA markers in the striatum with expression of parkinsonism.[76] This finding concurs with the finding in long-term MPTP monkeys with mild unilateral lesions.[35] These results suggest that decreased VMAT2 is a key pathogenic event that precedes nigrostriatal DA neuron degeneration. The loss of VMAT2 may result from an association with alpha-synuclein aggregation induced by oxidative stress.

Compensatory Mechanisms in PD

The longitudinal paradigm with DA-specific radioligands has also been used for PET imaging of compensatory mechanisms in PD.[3] A study of DA synthesis capacity in normal aging showed greater striatal uptake in older adults than in younger adults,[16] indicating possible compensation for deficits elsewhere in the DA system. A longitudinal study with 3 presynaptic DA markers of DA synthesis, DAT, and VMAT2 reported that younger patients with PD may have more efficient compensatory mechanisms.[77] At symptom onset, the loss of putamen DTBZ binding was substantially greater in younger compared with older patients with PD. However, the rate of DTBZ binding loss was significantly slower in younger patients. The estimated presymptomatic phase of the disease spanned more than 20 years in younger patients, compared with 10 years in older patients. These observations suggest that younger patients with PD progress more slowly and are able to endure more damage to the DA system before the appearance of first motor symptoms.

The age effects on disease progression revealed by DTBZ binding were absent in measures from FDOPA and DAT binding. The analysis of this dataset also yielded evidence for possible upregulation of DA synthesis and downregulation of DAT in the more severely affected putamen in the early stage of PD.[37] However, the normalized FDOPA and DAT binding values tended to approach VMAT2 binding values in the putamen in later stages of disease, when the rates of decline in the PET measures were similar for all the markers, suggesting that compensatory mechanisms decrease with the progression of PD.

Compensatory responses in intact monoamine neuron perikarya have also been examined by measuring extrastriatal FDOPA uptake.[75] Progressive loss in FDOPA uptake occurred in putamen (8.1%), locus coeruleus (7.8%), internal globus pallidus (7.7%), caudate (6.3%), and hypothalamus (6.1%). At baseline, levels of FDOPA uptake in internal pallidum and locus coeruleus increased in PD compared with controls, indicating possible compensatory upregulation. These increased levels normalized (internal pallidum) or became subnormal (locus coeruleus) at follow-up, suggesting exhaustion of compensation within the first years of disease. This finding agrees with an early cross-sectional study showing normal or increased FDOPA uptake in the substantia nigra, midbrain raphe, and locus coeruleus in early but not advanced PD.[48] The red nucleus, subthalamus, ventral thalamus, and pineal gland were also eventually involved. However, FDOPA uptake may also measure serotoninergic function in the median raphe nuclei complex, which has low or no DA innervation.[78] These studies show that loss of monoaminergic function in extrastriatal regions is delayed and occurs independently from nigrostriatal degeneration.

An increase of striatal DA D2 receptor binding has been reported with raclopride in patients with early untreated PD particularly in the putamen contralateral to the more affected body side (see **Fig. 3B**).[79] D2 receptor upregulation is evident in the striatum of human patients or animals with MPTP-induced parkinsonism. However, the initial upregulation in putamen may reverse with DA treatment, and increasing disease severity and binding values in the range of control subjects or lower may be encountered in patients with advanced PD. Because changes in raclopride binding and FDOPA uptake are associated throughout the disease course, it is likely that DA D2 receptor changes result from the decline in presynaptic DA drive.

In the study with FDOPA, MP, and DTBZ in long-term MPTP monkeys,[35] the decline in MP binding in the ventral striatum (−75%) exceeded the declines of DTBZ binding and FDOPA uptake in that region (−65%), suggesting that compensatory downmodulation of uptake sites may occur in the striatal regions with the least DA depletion. In the subacute unilateral MPTP model,[65] indices of striatal uptake of FDOPA, DAT, and VMAT2 correlated most strongly with each other, supporting a lack of differential regulation within 2 months after nigrostriatal injury. Another study reported that compensatory changes in nigrostriatal DA activity occurred in the recovered and parkinsonian monkeys when DA depletion was at least 88% of control,[64] which may be too late to explain compensatory mechanisms in the early asymptomatic period.

Evaluation of Antiparkinsonian Therapeutics

PET imaging with DA-specific radioligands has been successfully used to assess the therapeutic efficacy and possible complications of novel disease-modifying therapies, which is needed because clinical measures of disease severity may be subjected to placebo effects often present in neuropsychiatric patients participating in research trials. As an imaging marker, FDOPA uptake in the striatum is considered the gold standard (**Fig. 4**) in several open-label as well as double-blind, placebo-controlled clinical trials of striatal DA cell transplantation in patients with advanced PD (see Ref.[80]). It has been shown that clinical improvement after fetal DA tissue grafting is associated with increased FDOPA uptake in the transplanted putamen over a period of 4 to 15 years.[81,82] The efficacy of gene therapy has been evaluated in phase 1 trials using PET imaging with the AADC-specific radiotracer FMT. Short-term clinical improvement in the patients was related to increased FMT uptake up to 2 years after adeno-associated virus (AAV) vector-mediated gene delivery of AADC into the putamen of patients with PD.[83,84] The multitracer approach has proved to be useful in long-term follow-up studies after the implantation of fetal cells in patients with PD,[82] as well as retinal pigment epithelial cells and neural stem cells in nonhuman primate models of PD.[85,86] These studies show that increased FDOPA uptake is correlated with graft-induced DA release in the putamen measured by changes in raclopride binding.

It has been suggested that loss of DA nerve terminals in association with changes in postsynaptic DA receptors may underlie motor complications occurring in the course of treatment of PD. In

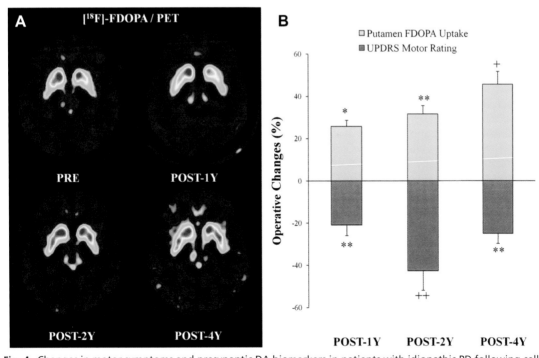

Fig. 4. Changes in motor symptoms and presynaptic DA biomarkers in patients with idiopathic PD following cell-based experimental therapies. (A) FDOPA PET images in one PD patient before (PRE) and 1 (POST-1Y), 2 (POST-2Y) and 4 (POST-4Y) years after fetal DA cell transplantation. (B) Decreased UPDRS motor ratings and increased FDOPA uptake in the putamen are observed at 1, 2, and 4 years in 15 patients with advanced PD following fetal DA cell transplantation. *P<.05, **P<.01, +P<.005, ++P<.0005. (*Data from* Ma Y, Peng S, Dhawan V, et al. Dopamine cell transplantation in Parkinson's disease: challenge and perspective. Br Med Bull 2011;100:177–9; with permission.)

patients with PD with and without dyskinesia, 1 hour after oral administration of levodopa/carbidopa,[87] levodopa-induced increases in synaptic DA levels in the striatum correlated positively with duration of PD symptoms. Patients with peak-dose dyskinesias had larger 1-hour increases in synaptic DA levels than stable responders, with no differences 4 hours after levodopa. Intermittent, large, levodopa-induced increases in synaptic DA concentration may lead to dramatic changes in receptor pharmacology and have been associated with the emergence of peak-dose dyskinesias in PD. In another study,[88] the putaminal DAT/VMAT2 binding ratio was decreased in patients with dyskinesia compared with those without dyskinesia. DAT downregulation may minimize symptoms by contributing to increased synaptic DA levels in early PD.

SUMMARY

PET studies have proved to be indispensable in providing information about PD using radioligands targeting nigrostriatal DA terminals. The development of presynaptic radiotracers for DA synthesis, DAT, and VMAT2 has led to viable means for imaging the nigrostriatal DA system. Some radiotracers binding to postsynaptic D2 receptors offer a quantitative approach to the measurement of endogenous DA release in relation to behavioral or pharmacologic stimulations. Many optimized imaging protocols and analytical methods are used to generate imaging biomarkers for clinical and research applications. The bulk of the work is focused on investigating the interaction between DA-specific lesions and impaired brain circuits that subserve motor and cognitive symptoms in PD. The results have provided new insights into the relationship between localized DA dysfunction and downstream effects within widely distributed functional brain networks over the course of disease onset and progression. This endeavor has led to advances in early differential diagnosis, in the understanding of molecular compensatory processes, and in the design of therapeutic trials in PD.

REFERENCES

1. Barrio JR, Huang SC, Phelps ME. Biological imaging and the molecular basis of dopaminergic diseases. Biochem Pharmacol 1997;54:341–8.

2. Stoessl AJ. Functional imaging studies of non-motoric manifestations of Parkinson's disease. Parkinsonism Relat Disord 2009;15(Suppl 3):S13–6.

3. Appel-Cresswell S, de la Fuente-Fernandez R, Galley S, et al. Imaging of compensatory mechanisms in Parkinson's disease. Curr Opin Neurol 2010;23:407–12.

4. Brooks DJ, Pavese N. Imaging biomarkers in Parkinson's disease. Prog Neurobiol 2011;95: 614–28.

5. Ma Y, Peng S, Dhawan V, et al. Cerebral glucose metabolism and blood flow in Parkinson's disease. In: Eidelberg D, editor. Imaging in Parkinson's disease. New York: Oxford University Press; 2011. p. 21–31.

6. Ma Y, Peng S, Spetsieris PG, et al. Abnormal metabolic brain networks in a nonhuman primate model of parkinsonism. J Cereb Blood Flow Metab 2012; 32:633–42.

7. Poston KL, Eidelberg D. FDG PET in the evaluation of Parkinson's disease. PET Clin 2010;5:55–64.

8. Huang SC, Yu DC, Barrio JR, et al. Kinetics and modeling of L-6-[18F]fluoro-dopa in human positron emission tomographic studies. J Cereb Blood Flow Metab 1991;11:898–913.

9. Cumming P, Leger GC, Kuwabara H, et al. Pharmacokinetics of plasma 6-[18F]fluoro-L-3,4-dihydroxy-phenylalanine ([18F]Fdopa) in humans. J Cereb Blood Flow Metab 1993;13:668–75.

10. Takikawa S, Dhawan V, Chaly T, et al. Input functions for 6-[fluorine-18]fluorodopa quantitation in parkinsonism: comparative studies and clinical correlations. J Nucl Med 1994;35:955–63.

11. Antonini A, Vontobel P, Psylla M, et al. Complementary positron emission tomographic studies of the striatal dopaminergic system in Parkinson's disease. Arch Neurol 1995;52:1183–90.

12. Sossi V, Doudet DJ, Holden JE. A reversible tracer analysis approach to the study of effective dopamine turnover. J Cereb Blood Flow Metab 2001; 21:469–76.

13. Melega WP, Grafton ST, Huang SC, et al. L-6-[18F] fluoro-dopa metabolism in monkeys and humans: biochemical parameters for the formulation of tracer kinetic models with positron emission tomography. J Cereb Blood Flow Metab 1991;11:890–7.

14. Yee RE, Huang SC, Stout DB, et al. Nigrostriatal reduction of aromatic L-amino acid decarboxylase activity in MPTP-treated squirrel monkeys: in vivo and in vitro investigations. J Neurochem 2000;74: 1147–57.

15. Barrio JR, Huang SC, Yu DC, et al. Radiofluorinated L-m-tyrosines: new in-vivo probes for central dopamine biochemistry. J Cereb Blood Flow Metab 1996;16:667–78.

16. Braskie MN, Wilcox CE, Landau SM, et al. Relationship of striatal dopamine synthesis capacity to age and cognition. J Neurosci 2008;28:14320–8.

17. Doudet DJ, Chan GL, Jivan S, et al. Evaluation of dopaminergic presynaptic integrity: 6-[18F] fluoro-L-dopa versus 6-[18F]fluoro-L-m-tyrosine. J Cereb Blood Flow Metab 1999;19:278–87.

18. Yagi S, Yoshikawa E, Futatsubashi M, et al. Progression from unilateral to bilateral parkinsonism in early Parkinson disease: implication of mesocortical dopamine dysfunction by PET. J Nucl Med 2010;51:1250–7.

19. Lotze M, Reimold M, Heymans U, et al. Reduced ventrolateral fMRI response during observation of emotional gestures related to the degree of dopaminergic impairment in Parkinson disease. J Cogn Neurosci 2009;21:1321–31.

20. Wang J, Zuo CT, Jiang YP, et al. 18F-FP-CIT PET imaging and SPM analysis of dopamine transporters in Parkinson's disease in various Hoehn & Yahr stages. J Neurol 2007;254:185–90.

21. Ravina B, Marek K, Eberly S, et al. Dopamine transporter imaging is associated with long-term outcomes in Parkinson's disease. Mov Disord 2012; 27:1392–7.

22. Eshuis SA, Jager PL, Maguire RP, et al. Direct comparison of FP-CIT SPECT and F-DOPA PET in patients with Parkinson's disease and healthy controls. Eur J Nucl Med Mol Imaging 2009;36: 454–62.

23. Fernagut PO, Li Q, Dovero S, et al. Dopamine transporter binding is unaffected by L-DOPA administration in normal and MPTP-treated monkeys. PLoS One 2010;5:e14053.

24. Bohnen NI, Albin RL, Koeppe RA, et al. Positron emission tomography of monoaminergic vesicular binding in aging and Parkinson disease. J Cereb Blood Flow Metab 2006;26:1198–212.

25. Zhu L, Liu Y, Plossl K, et al. An improved radiosynthesis of [18F]AV-133: a PET imaging agent for vesicular monoamine transporter 2. Nucl Med Biol 2010;37:133–41.

26. Frey KA, Koeppe RA, Kilbourn MR, et al. Presynaptic monoaminergic vesicles in Parkinson's disease and normal aging. Ann Neurol 1996;40: 873–84.

27. Tong J, Boileau I, Furukawa Y, et al. Distribution of vesicular monoamine transporter 2 protein in human brain: implications for brain imaging studies. J Cereb Blood Flow Metab 2011;31:2065–75.

28. Ko JH, Ptito A, Monchi O, et al. Increased dopamine release in the right anterior cingulate cortex during the performance of a sorting task: a [11C]FLB 457 PET study. Neuroimage 2009;46: 516–21.

29. Ceccarini J, Vrieze E, Koole M, et al. Optimized in vivo detection of dopamine release using 18F-fallypride PET. J Nucl Med 2012;53:1565–72.

30. Koepp MJ, Gunn RN, Lawrence AD, et al. Evidence for striatal dopamine release during a video game. Nature 1998;393:266–8.

31. Sawamoto N, Piccini P, Hotton G, et al. Cognitive deficits and striato-frontal dopamine release in Parkinson's disease. Brain 2008;131:1294–302.

32. Piccini P, Pavese N, Brooks DJ. Endogenous dopamine release after pharmacological challenges in Parkinson's disease. Ann Neurol 2003;53:647–53.

33. Slifstein M, Kegeles LS, Xu X, et al. Striatal and extrastriatal dopamine release measured with PET and [(18)F] fallypride. Synapse 2010;64:350–62.

34. Volkow ND, Wang GJ, Fowler JS, et al. Parallel loss of presynaptic and postsynaptic dopamine markers in normal aging. Ann Neurol 1998;44: 143–7.

35. Doudet DJ, Rosa-Neto P, Munk OL, et al. Effect of age on markers for monoaminergic neurons of normal and MPTP-lesioned rhesus monkeys: a multi-tracer PET study. Neuroimage 2006;30:26–35.

36. Lee CS, Samii A, Sossi V, et al. In vivo positron emission tomographic evidence for compensatory changes in presynaptic dopaminergic nerve terminals in Parkinson's disease. Ann Neurol 2000;47: 493–503.

37. Nandhagopal R, Kuramoto L, Schulzer M, et al. Longitudinal evolution of compensatory changes in striatal dopamine processing in Parkinson's disease. Brain 2011;134:3290–8.

38. Patlak CS, Blasberg RG, Fenstermacher JD. Graphical evaluation of blood-to-brain transfer constants from multiple-time uptake data. J Cereb Blood Flow Metab 1983;3:1–7.

39. Logan J. Graphical analysis of PET data applied to reversible and irreversible tracers. Nucl Med Biol 2000;27:661–70 [Record as supplied by publisher].

40. Gunn RN, Lammertsma AA, Hume SP, et al. Parametric imaging of ligand-receptor binding in PET using a simplified reference region model. Neuroimage 1997;6:279–87.

41. Sossi V, Holden JE, Chan G, et al. Analysis of four dopaminergic tracers kinetics using two different tissue input function methods. J Cereb Blood Flow Metab 2000;20:653–60.

42. Ichise M, Liow JS, Lu JQ, et al. Linearized reference tissue parametric imaging methods: application to [11C]DASB positron emission tomography studies of the serotonin transporter in human brain. J Cereb Blood Flow Metab 2003;23:1096–112.

43. Dhawan V, Ma Y, Pillai V, et al. Comparative analysis of striatal FDOPA uptake in Parkinson's disease: ratio method versus graphical approach. J Nucl Med 2002;43:1324–30.

44. Jokinen P, Helenius H, Rauhala E, et al. Simple ratio analysis of 18F-fluorodopa uptake in striatal subregions separates patients with early Parkinson disease from healthy controls. J Nucl Med 2009;50: 893–9.

45. Lin KJ, Lin WY, Hsieh CJ, et al. Optimal scanning time window for 18F-FP-(+)-DTBZ (18F-AV-133) summed uptake measurements. Nucl Med Biol 2011;38:1149–55.

46. Panzacchi A, Moresco RM, Garibotto V, et al. A voxel-based PET study of dopamine transporters in Parkinson's disease: relevance of age at onset. Neurobiol Dis 2008;31:102–9.

47. Okamura N, Villemagne VL, Drago J, et al. In vivo measurement of vesicular monoamine transporter type 2 density in Parkinson disease with (18)F-AV-133. J Nucl Med 2010;51:223–8.

48. Moore RY, Whone AL, Brooks DJ. Extrastriatal monoamine neuron function in Parkinson's disease: an 18F-dopa PET study. Neurobiol Dis 2008;29:381–90.

49. Lewis SJ, Pavese N, Rivero-Bosch M, et al. Brain monoamine systems in multiple system atrophy: a positron emission tomography study. Neurobiol Dis 2012;46:130–6.

50. Oh M, Kim JS, Kim JY, et al. Subregional patterns of preferential striatal dopamine transporter loss differ in Parkinson disease, progressive supranuclear palsy, and multiple-system atrophy. J Nucl Med 2012;53:399–406.

51. la Fougere C, Popperl G, Levin J, et al. The value of the dopamine D2/3 receptor ligand 18F-desmethoxyfallypride for the differentiation of idiopathic and nonidiopathic parkinsonian syndromes. J Nucl Med 2010;51:581–7.

52. Eckert T, Feigin A, Lewis DE, et al. Regional metabolic changes in parkinsonian patients with normal dopaminergic imaging. Mov Disord 2007;22:167–73.

53. Silveira-Moriyama L, Schwingenschuh P, O'Donnell A, et al. Olfaction in patients with suspected parkinsonism and scans without evidence of dopaminergic deficit (SWEDDs). J Neurol Neurosurg Psychiatry 2009;80:744–8.

54. Schneider SA, Edwards MJ, Mir P, et al. Patients with adult-onset dystonic tremor resembling parkinsonian tremor have scans without evidence of dopaminergic deficit (SWEDDs). Mov Disord 2007;22:2210–5.

55. Sudmeyer M, Antke C, Zizek T, et al. Diagnostic accuracy of combined FP-CIT, IBZM, and MIBG scintigraphy in the differential diagnosis of degenerative parkinsonism: a multidimensional statistical approach. J Nucl Med 2011;52:733–40.

56. Adams JR, van Netten H, Schulzer M, et al. PET in LRRK2 mutations: comparison to sporadic Parkinson's disease and evidence for presymptomatic compensation. Brain 2005;128:2777–85.

57. Ribeiro MJ, Thobois S, Lohmann E, et al. A multitracer dopaminergic PET study of young-onset parkinsonian patients with and without parkin gene mutations. J Nucl Med 2009;50:1244–50.

58. Eggers C, Schmidt A, Hagenah J, et al. Progression of subtle motor signs in PINK1 mutation carriers with mild dopaminergic deficit. Neurology 2010;74:1798–805.

59. Gallagher CL, Oakes TR, Johnson SC, et al. Rate of 6-[18F]fluorodopa uptake decline in striatal subregions in Parkinson's disease. Mov Disord 2011;26:614–20.

60. van Beilen M, Portman AT, Kiers HA, et al. Striatal FDOPA uptake and cognition in advanced non-demented Parkinson's disease: a clinical and FDOPA-PET study. Parkinsonism Relat Disord 2008;14:224–8.

61. Polito C, Berti V, Ramat S, et al. Interaction of caudate dopamine depletion and brain metabolic changes with cognitive dysfunction in early Parkinson's disease. Neurobiol Aging 2012;33:206. e229–39.

62. Niethammer M, Tang CC, Ma Y, et al. Parkinson's disease cognitive network correlates with caudate dopamine. Neuroimage 2013;78:204–9.

63. Yee RE, Irwin I, Milonas C, et al. Novel observations with FDOPA-PET imaging after early nigrostriatal damage. Mov Disord 2001;16:838–48.

64. Blesa J, Pifl C, Sanchez-Gonzalez MA, et al. The nigrostriatal system in the presymptomatic and symptomatic stages in the MPTP monkey model: a PET, histological and biochemical study. Neurobiol Dis 2012;48:79–91.

65. Karimi M, Tian L, Brown CA, et al. Validation of nigrostriatal positron emission tomography measures: critical limits. Ann Neurol 2013;73:390–6.

66. de la Fuente-Fernandez R, Lu JQ, Sossi V, et al. Biochemical variations in the synaptic level of dopamine precede motor fluctuations in Parkinson's disease: PET evidence of increased dopamine turnover. Ann Neurol 2001;49:298–303.

67. de la Fuente-Fernandez R, Ruth TJ, Sossi V, et al. Expectation and dopamine release: mechanism of the placebo effect in Parkinson's disease. Science 2001;293:1164–6.

68. Steeves TD, Miyasaki J, Zurowski M, et al. Increased striatal dopamine release in Parkinsonian patients with pathological gambling: a [11C] raclopride PET study. Brain 2009;132:1376–85.

69. Ray NJ, Miyasaki JM, Zurowski M, et al. Extrastriatal dopaminergic abnormalities of DA homeostasis in Parkinson's patients with medication-induced pathological gambling: a [11C] FLB-457 and PET study. Neurobiol Dis 2012;48:519–25.

70. Nandhagopal R, Mak E, Schulzer M, et al. Progression of dopaminergic dysfunction in a LRRK2 kindred: a multitracer PET study. Neurology 2008; 71:1790–5.

71. Huang C, Tang C, Feigin A, et al. Changes in network activity with the progression of Parkinson's disease. Brain 2007;130:1834–46.

72. Tang CC, Poston KL, Dhawan V, et al. Abnormalities in metabolic network activity precede the onset of motor symptoms in Parkinson's disease. J Neurosci 2010;30:1049–56.

73. Bruck A, Aalto S, Rauhala E, et al. A follow-up study on 6-[18F]fluoro-L-dopa uptake in early

Parkinson's disease shows nonlinear progression in the putamen. Mov Disord 2009;24:1009–15.

74. Nandhagopal R, Kuramoto L, Schulzer M, et al. Longitudinal progression of sporadic Parkinson's disease: a multi-tracer positron emission tomography study. Brain 2009;132:2970–9.

75. Pavese N, Rivero-Bosch M, Lewis SJ, et al. Progression of monoaminergic dysfunction in Parkinson's disease: a longitudinal 18F-dopa PET study. Neuroimage 2011;56:1463–8.

76. Chen MK, Kuwabara H, Zhou Y, et al. VMAT2 and dopamine neuron loss in a primate model of Parkinson's disease. J Neurochem 2008;105:78–90.

77. de la Fuente-Fernandez R, Schulzer M, Kuramoto L, et al. Age-specific progression of nigrostriatal dysfunction in Parkinson's disease. Ann Neurol 2011;69:803–10.

78. Pavese N, Simpson BS, Metta V, et al. [18F]FDOPA uptake in the raphe nuclei complex reflects serotonin transporter availability. A combined [18F]FDOPA and [11C]DASB PET study in Parkinson's disease. Neuroimage 2012;59:1080–4.

79. Rinne JO, Laihinen A, Ruottinen H, et al. Increased density of dopamine D2 receptors in the putamen, but not in the caudate nucleus in early Parkinson's disease: a PET study with [11C]raclopride. J Neurol Sci 1995;132:156–61.

80. Ma Y, Peng S, Dhawan V, et al. Dopamine cell transplantation in Parkinson's disease: challenge and perspective. Br Med Bull 2011;100:173–89.

81. Ma Y, Tang C, Chaly T, et al. Dopamine cell implantation in Parkinson's disease: long-term clinical and (18)F-FDOPA PET outcomes. J Nucl Med 2010;51:7–15.

82. Politis M, Wu K, Loane C, et al. Serotonin neuron loss and nonmotor symptoms continue in Parkinson's patients treated with dopamine grafts. Sci Transl Med 2012;4:128ra41.

83. Christine CW, Starr PA, Larson PS, et al. Safety and tolerability of putaminal AADC gene therapy for Parkinson disease. Neurology 2009;73:1662–9.

84. Muramatsu S, Fujimoto K, Kato S, et al. A phase I study of aromatic L-amino acid decarboxylase gene therapy for Parkinson's disease. Mol Ther 2010;18:1731–5.

85. Doudet DJ, Cornfeldt ML, Honey CR, et al. PET imaging of implanted human retinal pigment epithelial cells in the MPTP-induced primate model of Parkinson's disease. Exp Neurol 2004;189:361–8.

86. Muramatsu S, Okuno T, Suzuki Y, et al. Multitracer assessment of dopamine function after transplantation of embryonic stem cell-derived neural stem cells in a primate model of Parkinson's disease. Synapse 2009;63:541–8.

87. de la Fuente-Fernandez R, Sossi V, Huang Z, et al. Levodopa-induced changes in synaptic dopamine levels increase with progression of Parkinson's disease: implications for dyskinesias. Brain 2004;127:2747–54.

88. Troiano AR, de la Fuente-Fernandez R, Sossi V, et al. PET demonstrates reduced dopamine transporter expression in PD with dyskinesias. Neurology 2009;72:1211–6.

Index

Note: Page numbers of article titles are in **boldface** type.

PET Clin 8 (2013) 487–490
http://dx.doi.org/10.1016/S1556-8598(13)00087-4
1556-8598/13/$ – see front matter © 2013 Elsevier Inc. All rights reserved.

pet.theclinics.com

Moving?

Make sure your subscription moves with you!

To notify us of your new address, find your **Clinics Account Number** (located on your mailing label above your name), and contact customer service at:

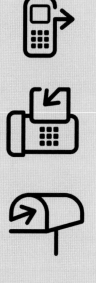

Email: journalscustomerservice-usa@elsevier.com

800-654-2452 (subscribers in the U.S. & Canada)
314-447-8871 (subscribers outside of the U.S. & Canada)

Fax number: 314-447-8029

Elsevier Health Sciences Division
Subscription Customer Service
3251 Riverport Lane
Maryland Heights, MO 63043

*To ensure uninterrupted delivery of your subscription, please notify us at least 4 weeks in advance of move.